Lymphedema Diet Cookbook

49+ Super Tasty Lymphedema Recipes to Try Out Today!

BY - Alain Duke

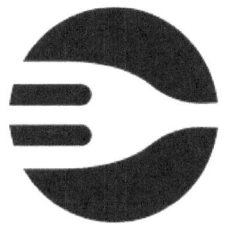

Copyright Notification

Table of Contents

Introduction:

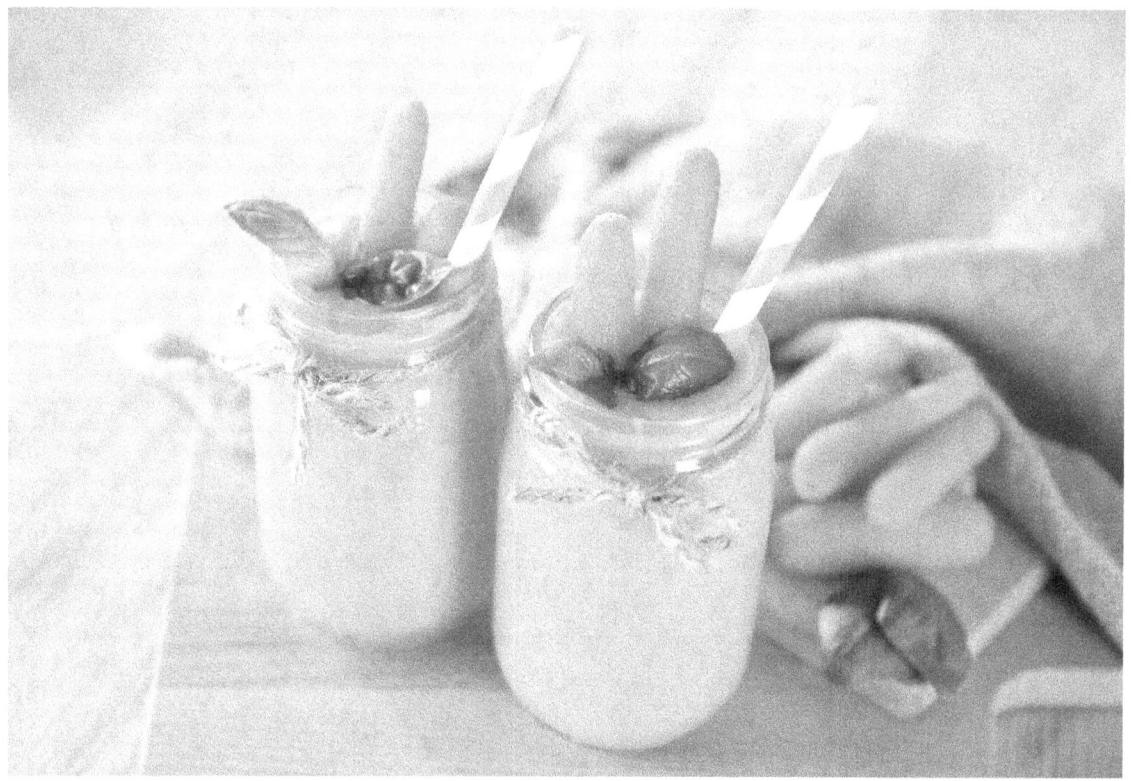

Do you ever find yourself wondering how to enhance your well-being through the power of nutrition? Are you searching for delicious recipes that not only tantalize your taste buds but also support your health journey? If you or someone you know is navigating the challenges of lymphedema, you're likely aware of the importance of a mindful diet. What if you could embark on a culinary adventure designed to both delight your palate and contribute to your overall wellness?

As you dive into these pages, you'll discover a treasure trove of culinary inspiration that extends far beyond bland and restrictive diets. Imagine savoring mouthwatering dishes that not only meet your nutritional needs but also make mealtime an experience to look forward to. Whether you're a seasoned chef or just finding your way around the kitchen, these recipes are crafted to be accessible, enjoyable, and, most importantly, beneficial for managing lymphedema.

So, are you ready to embark on a culinary adventure that not only satisfies your taste buds but also contributes to your well-being? This cookbook is more than a collection of recipes; it's your guide to transforming the way you eat for a healthier, more flavorful life.

Don't just read about it – experience it for yourself! Turn the page, start cooking, and let the journey to better lymphatic health begin. Your body will thank you, one delicious bite at a time.

Chapter 1: Breakfast Recipes

1. Apple Pancakes

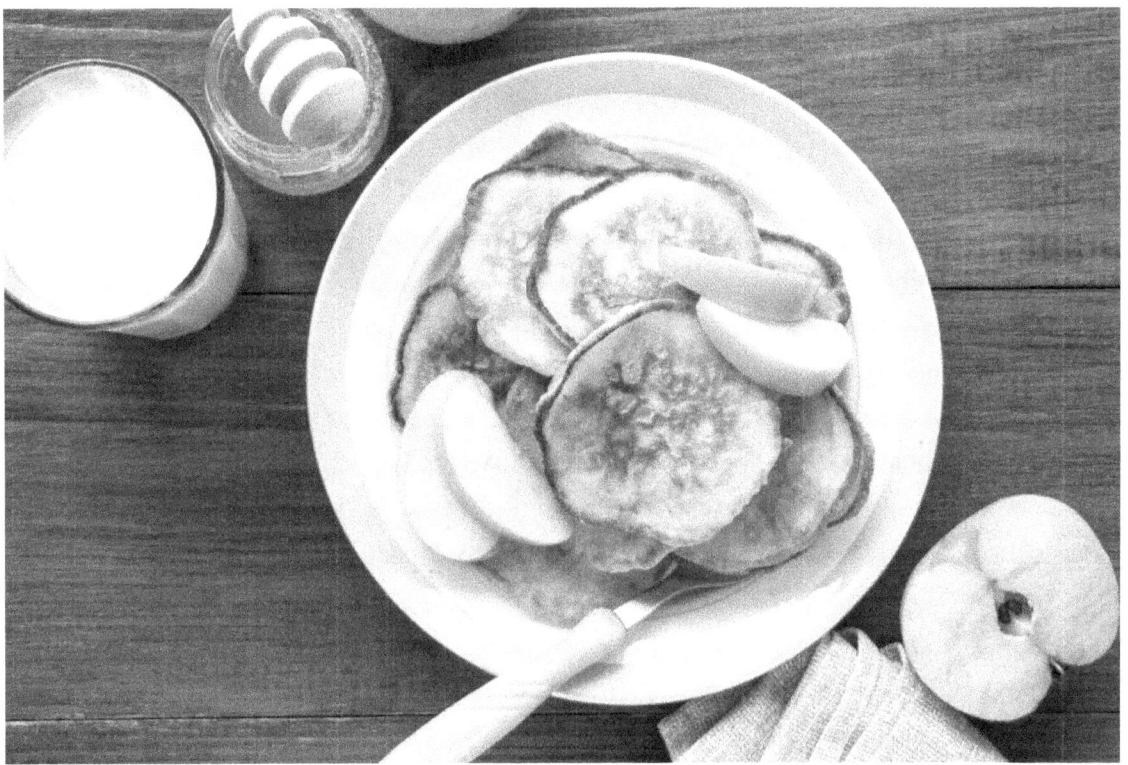

Packed with vitamins and antioxidants, these pancakes offer a guilt-free treat for all ages. Easy to prepare and versatile, they cater to diverse dietary preferences, making mornings a flavorful and health-conscious affair.

Cooking time: 15 minutes

Servings: 4

Ingredients:

- 1 cup whole wheat flour
- ¼ tsp baking soda
- ¼ tsp baking powder
- 1 cup apples, chopped
- 2 eggs
- 1 cup milk

Instructions:

In a bowl, combine all ingredients together and mix well.

In a skillet, heat olive oil, pour ¼ of the batter and cook each pancake for 1-2 minutes per side.

When ready, remove from heat and serve.

2. Peach Pecan Pie

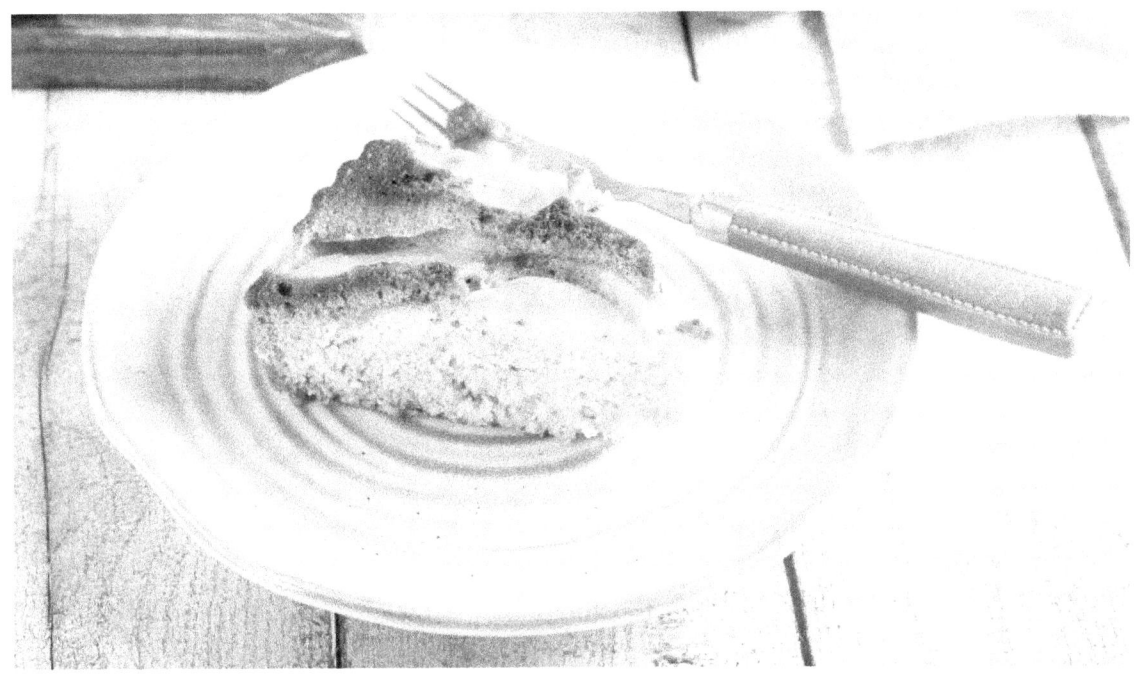

This wholesome meal is a nutritional gem, rich in antioxidants, fiber, and heart-healthy fats. Perfect for gatherings or a sweet family treat, it caters to all taste buds while providing a guilt-free, naturally sweetened experience.

Cooking time: 45 minutes

Servings: 8

Ingredients:

- 4-5 cups peaches
- 1 tablespoon preserves
- 1 cup sugar
- 4 small egg yolks
- ¼ cup flour
- 1 tsp vanilla extract

Instructions:

Line a pie plate or pie form with pastry and cover the edges of the plate depending on your preference.

In a bowl, combine all pie ingredients together and mix well.

Pour the mixture over the pastry.

Bake at 400-425 F for 25-30 minutes or until golden brown.

When ready, remove from the oven and let it rest for 15 minutes.

3. Breakfast Casserole

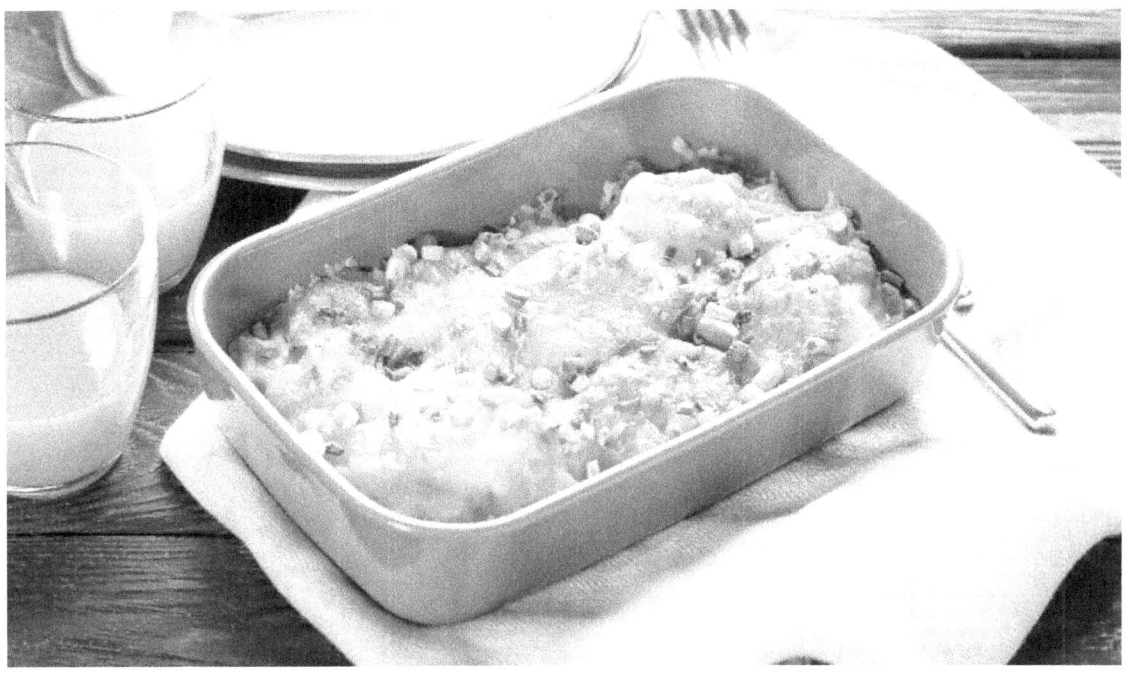

This easy-to-make dish suits various dietary preferences, making it a versatile choice for families and individuals alike.

Cooking time: 45 minutes

Servings: 4

Ingredients:

- 1 can crescent rolls
- 1 lb. bacon
- 1 cup cheddar cheese
- 4 eggs
- ¼ cup almond milk
- ¼ tsp salt

Instructions:

Sprinkle bacon and cheese.

In a bowl, whisk eggs and milk together.

Pour mixture over the cheese mixture.

Bake at 350 F for 28-30 minutes.

When ready, remove from heat and serve.

4. Gingerbread Muffins

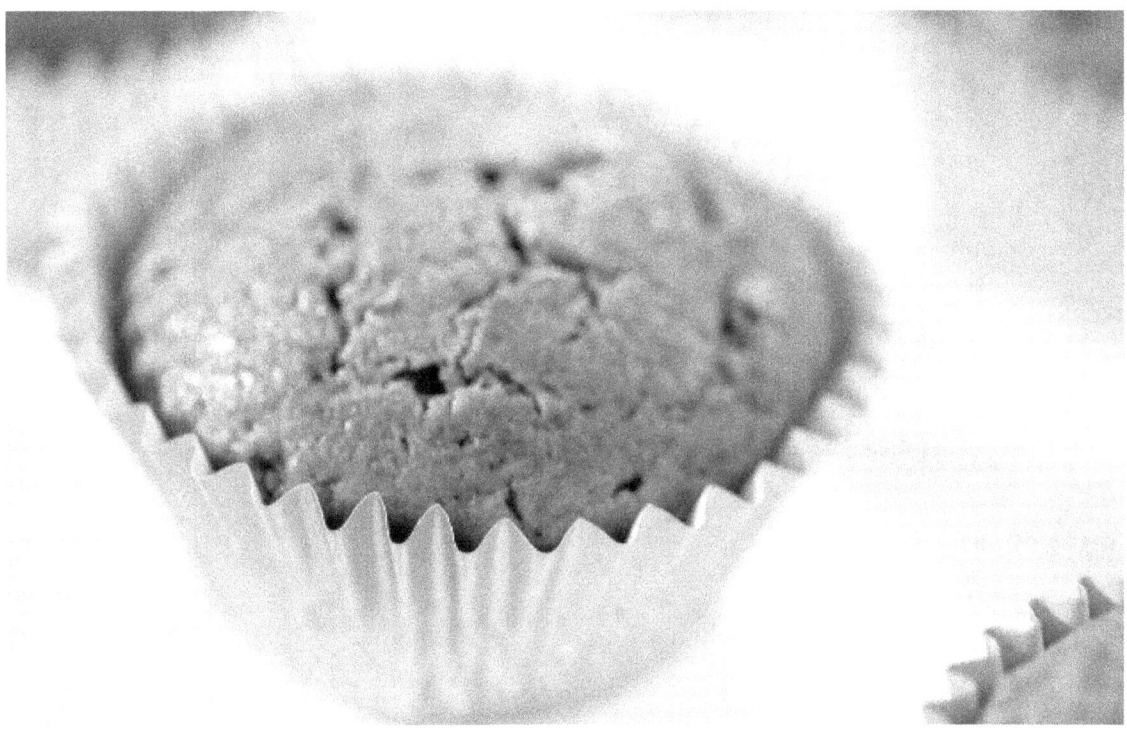

Wholesome and warmly spiced, the gingerbread muffins effortlessly blend the nostalgic aroma of ginger, cinnamon, and molasses.

Cooking time: 30 minutes

Servings: 10

Ingredients:

- 2 eggs
- 1 tablespoon olive oil
- 1 cup milk
- 2 cups whole wheat flour
- 1 tsp baking soda
- ¼ tsp baking soda
- 1 tsp ginger
- 1 tsp cinnamon
- ¼ cup molasses

Instructions:

In a bowl, combine all dry ingredients.

In another bowl, combine all dry ingredients.

Combine wet and dry ingredients together.

Fold in ginger and mix well.

Pour mixture into 8-12 prepared muffin cups, fill 2/3 of the cups.

Bake for 18-20 minutes at 375 F.

When ready, remove from the oven and serve.

5. Avocado Toast

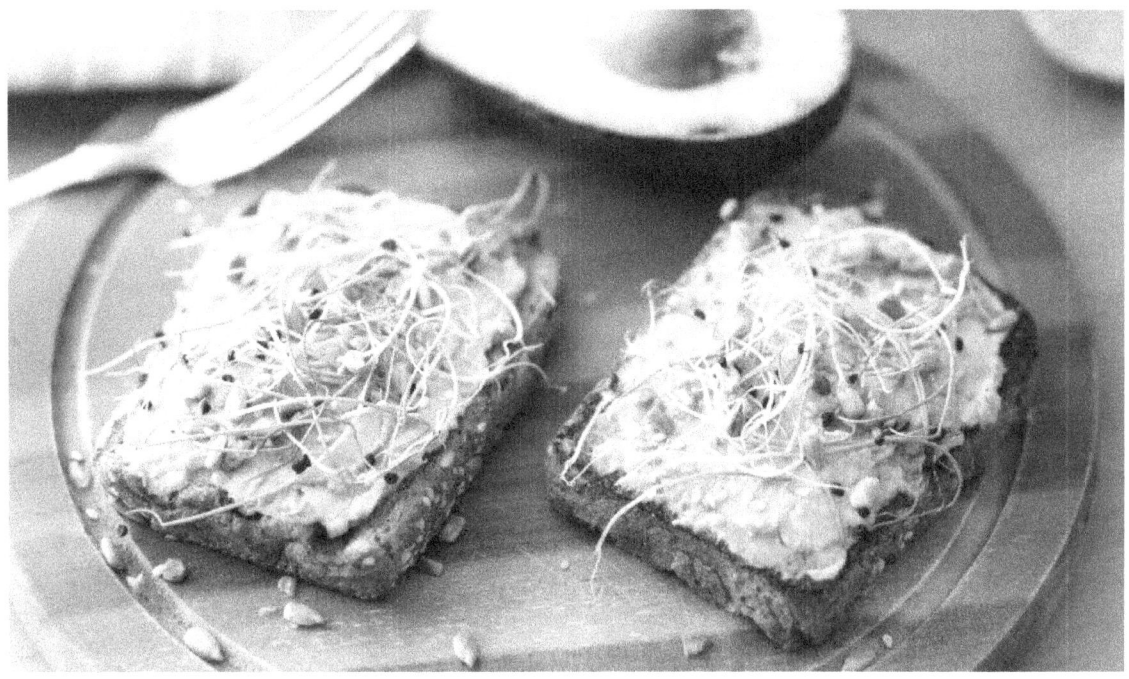

Packed with heart-healthy fats and anti-inflammatory properties, avocados aid in reducing swelling. This versatile dish suits all taste buds, offering a perfect balance of flavors and textures.

Cooking time: 10 minutes

Servings: 2

Ingredients:

- 2 slices bread
- ½ avocado
- 2 tablespoons hemp seeds
- ¼ tsp pepper

Instructions:

Toast the bread slices.

Mass the avocado and spread on the bread.

Top with hemp seeds and a dash of pepper.

Serve when ready.

6. Bok Choy Omelette

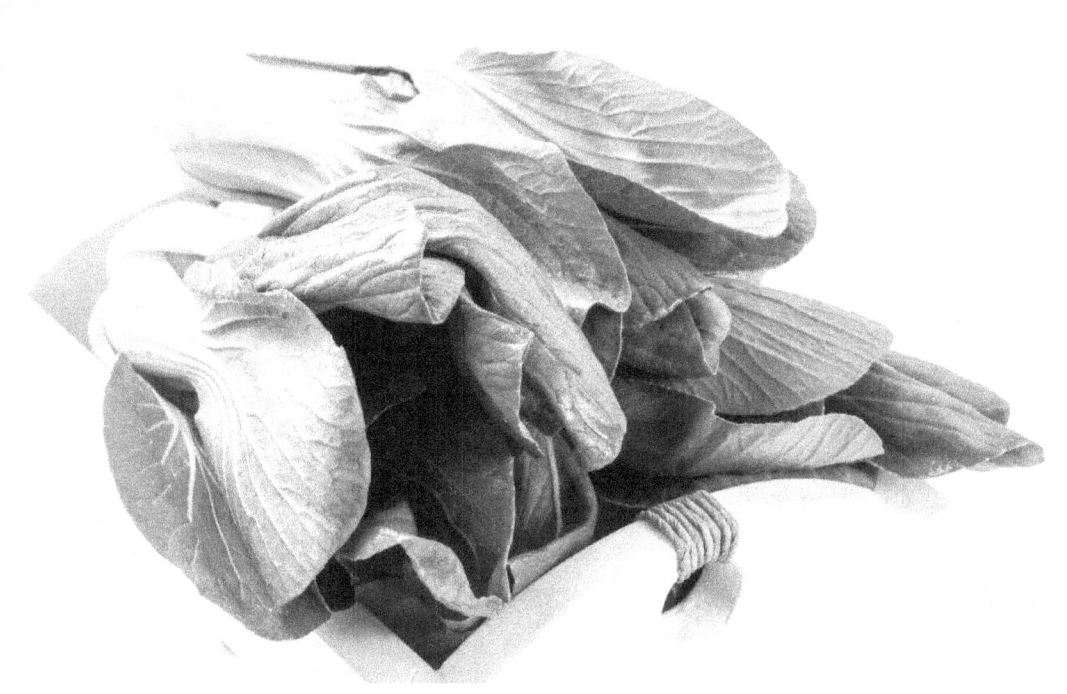

Nourish your body with our Lymphedema-Friendly Bok Choy Omelette, a nutrient-packed delight. Packed with anti-inflammatory properties from fresh Bok choy, this recipe is tailored for lymphedema patients.

Cooking time: 15 minutes

Servings: 1

Ingredients:

- 2 eggs
- ¼ tsp salt
- ¼ tsp black pepper
- 1 tablespoon olive oil
- ¼ cup cheese
- ¼ tsp basil
- 1 cup bok choy

Instructions:

In a bowl, combine all ingredients together and mix well.

In a skillet, heat olive oil and pour the egg mixture.

Cook for 1-2 minutes per side.

When ready, remove omelette from the skillet and serve.

7. Kiwi Pancakes

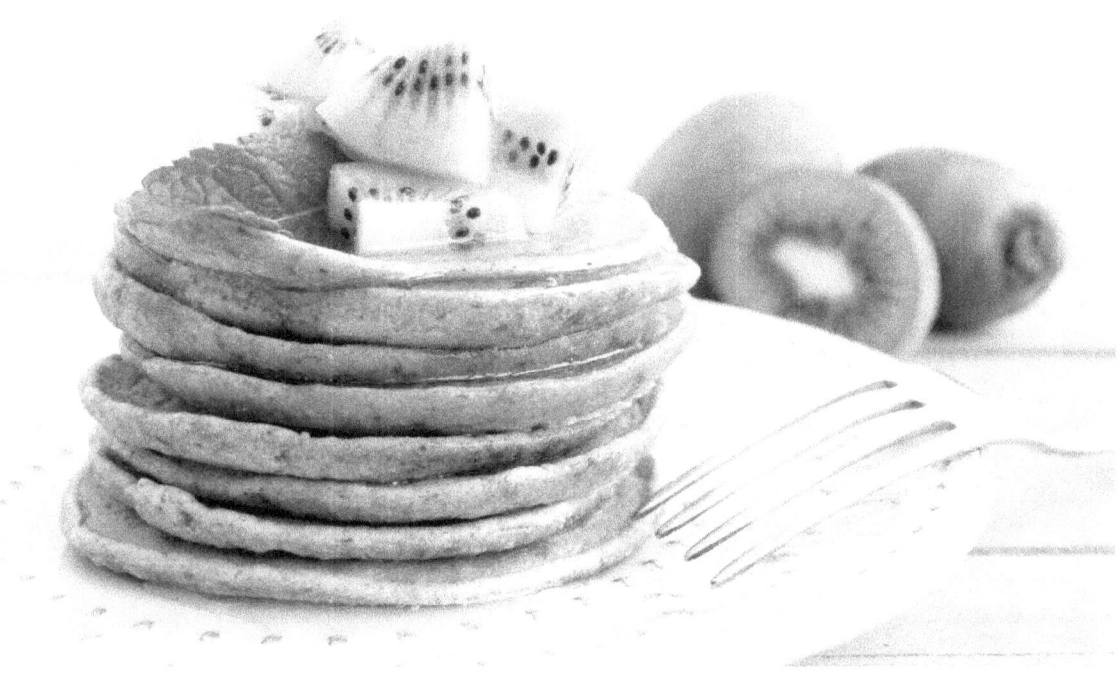

These delectable pancakes are not only delicious but also packed with health benefits. Kiwis are loaded with vitamins and antioxidants, promoting immune health and aiding digestion. Plus, these pancakes are suitable for all dietary preferences, making them a delightful and inclusive breakfast option for everyone.

Cooking time: 30 minutes

Servings: 4

Ingredients:

- 1 cup whole wheat flour
- ¼ tsp baking soda
- ¼ tsp baking powder
- 1 cup mashed kiwi
- 2 eggs
- 1 cup milk

Instructions:

In a bowl, combine all ingredients together and mix well.

In a skillet, heat olive oil.

Pour ¼ of the batter and cook each pancake for 1-2 minutes per side.

When ready, remove from heat and serve.

8. Spinach Omelette

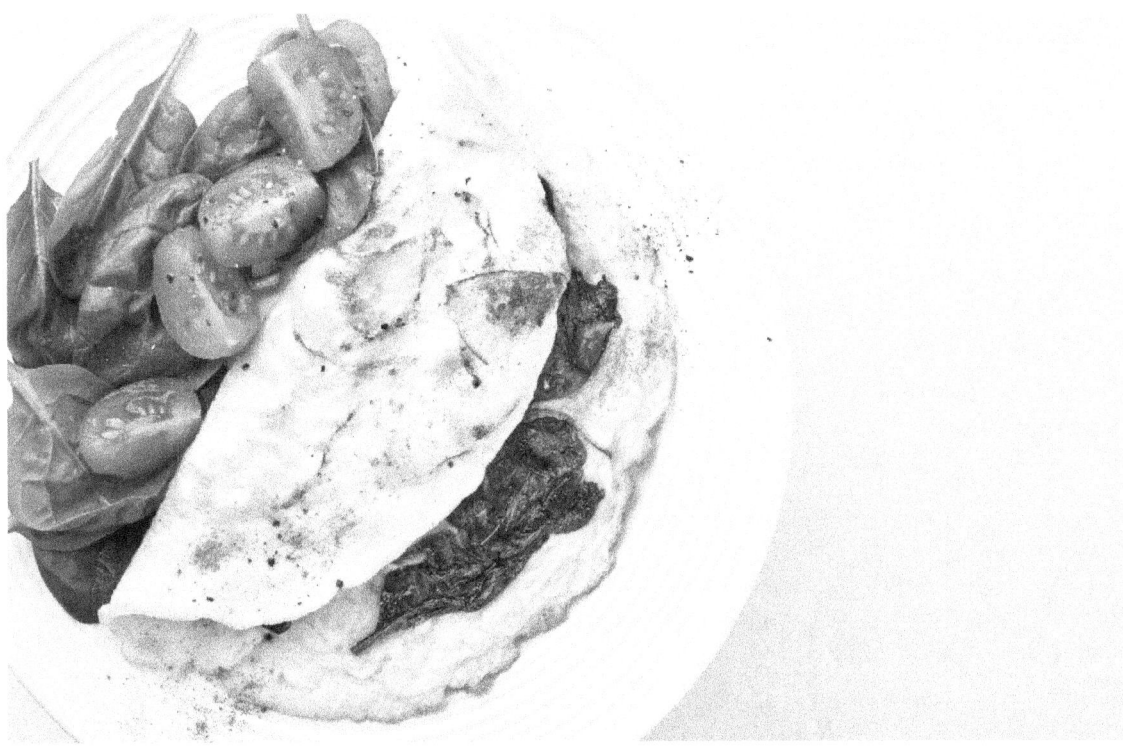

Packed with lean protein and enriched with spinach, this dish supports a healthy lifestyle. The low sodium content ensures suitability for all, promoting overall well-being. Embrace a flavorful solution that prioritizes your health without compromising on taste—a wholesome choice for those managing lymphedema.

Cooking time: 15 minutes

Servings: 1

Ingredients:

- 2 eggs
- ¼ tsp salt
- ¼ tsp black pepper
- 1 tablespoon olive oil
- ¼ cup cheese
- ¼ tsp basil
- 1 cup spinach

Instructions:

In a bowl, combine all ingredients together and mix well.

In a skillet, heat olive oil and pour the egg mixture.

Cook for 1-2 minutes per side.

When ready, remove omelette from the skillet and serve.

9. Pear Muffins

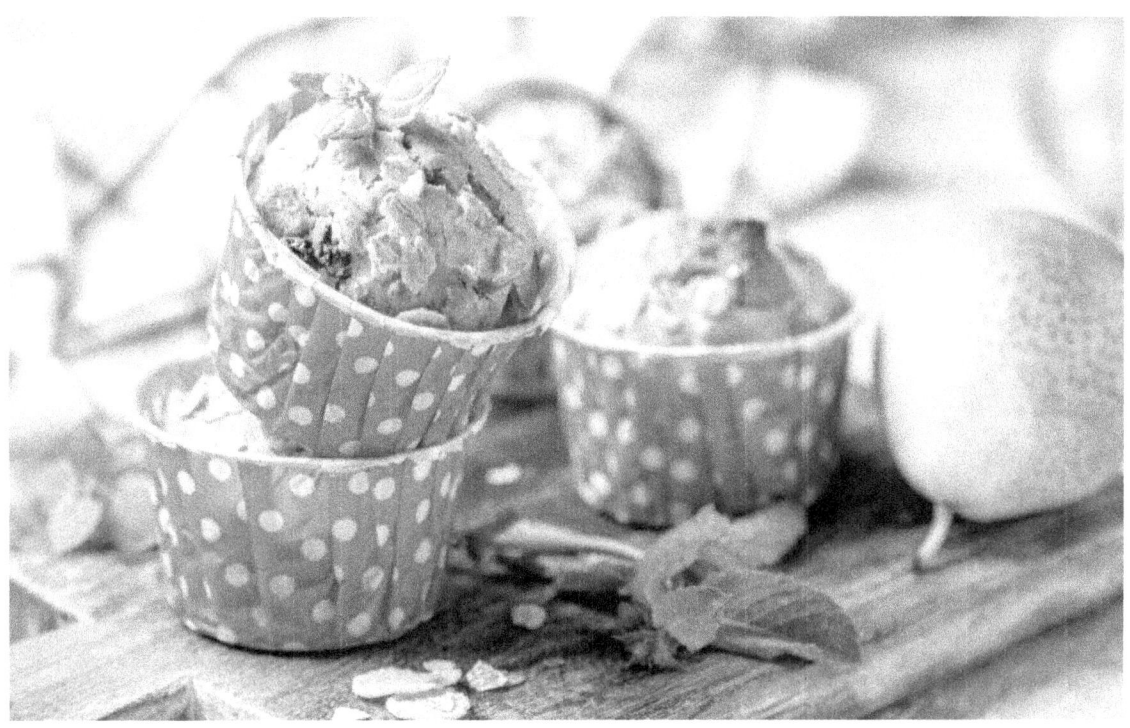

These delectable Pear Muffins offer a delightful twist to your morning routine. Bursting with the goodness of fresh pears, they provide a wholesome way to start your day.

Cooking time: 30 minutes

Servings: 10

Ingredients:

- 2 eggs
- 1 tablespoon olive oil
- 1 cup milk
- 2 cups whole wheat flour
- 1 tsp baking soda
- ¼ tsp baking soda
- 1 tsp cinnamon
- 1 cup mashed pear

Instructions:

In a bowl, combine all dry ingredients.

In another bowl, combine all dry ingredients.

Combine wet and dry ingredients together.

Pour mixture into 8-12 prepared muffin cups, fill 2/3 of the cups.

Bake for 18-20 minutes at 375 F.

When ready, remove from the oven and serve.

10. Breakfast Potatoes

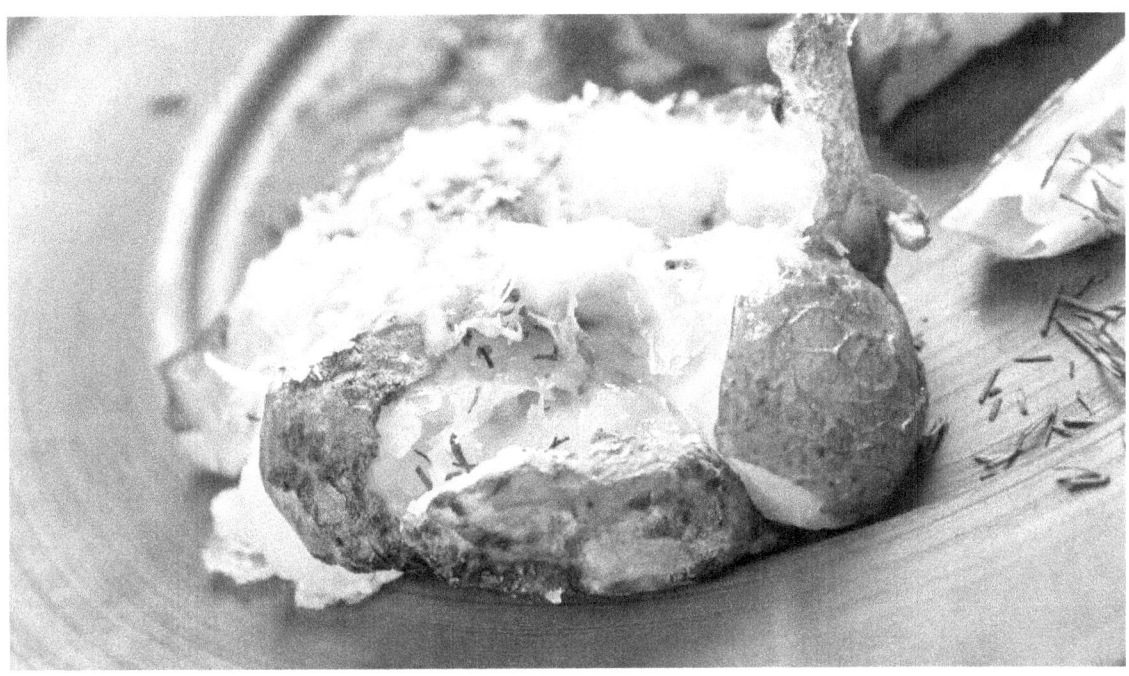

Start your day right with our nutritious Breakfast Potatoes, a lymphedema-friendly recipe packed with essential nutrients. These carefully crafted potatoes provide a satisfying, energy-boosting meal without compromising on taste.

Cooking time: 30 minutes

Servings: 4

Ingredients:

- 2 potatoes
- 2 tablespoons olive oil
- 1 pinch salt
- 1 tablespoon parmesan cheese

Instructions:

In a skillet, heat olive oil.

Add slices of potatoes and fry on low heat.

Sprinkle with salt and cook until the potatoes are brown.

When ready, transfer to a plate and sprinkle parmesan cheese and serve.

Chapter 2: Main course Recipes

11. Swedish Meatballs

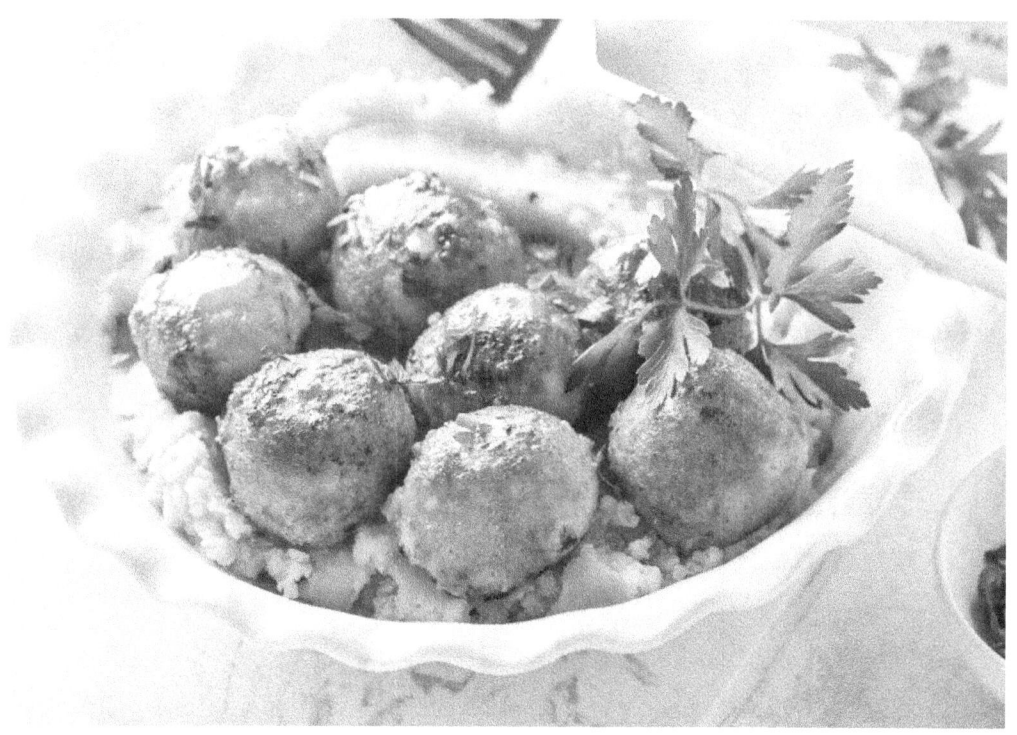

Discover a lymphedema-friendly delight with Swedish Meatballs. Crafted with lean meats and wholesome ingredients, this recipe champions a low-sodium, anti-inflammatory approach.

Cooking time: 30 minutes

Servings: 6

Ingredients:

- 1 cup sunflower oil
- ¼ cup coconut milk
- 1 tsp onion powder
- 1 tsp
- salt
- 4 lbs. ground beef
- 2 eggs
- 1 tsp black pepper
- ¼ tsp allspice
- ¼ tsp nutmeg

Sauce:

- ½ cup butter
- ¼ cup parmesan cheese
- 5 cups beef broth
- ¼ cup coconut milk
- ¼ tsp salt

Instructions:

Preheat the oven to 375 F.

In a bowl, mix all meatballs ingredients using a stand mixer.

Form little balls and bake for 20-25 minutes or until done.

In a skillet, sauce parmesan cheese, whisk in beef broth, salt, and coconut milk, cook until thickened.

Serve on top of meatballs.

12. Asparagus Frittata

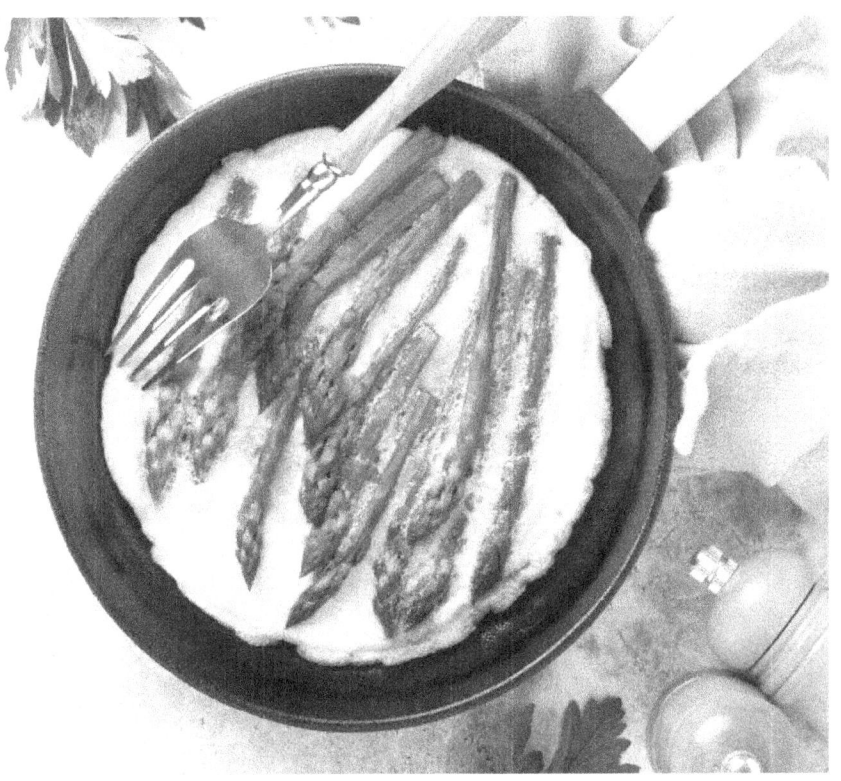

The Asparagus Frittata is a wholesome and nutritious dish that's both delicious and health-conscious. Packed with fresh asparagus, eggs, and a medley of flavorful ingredients, this recipe offers a low-calorie, high-fiber option for anyone looking to maintain a balanced diet.

Cooking time: 30 minutes

Servings: 2

Ingredients:

- ½ lb. asparagus
- 1 tablespoon olive oil
- ½ red onion
- 2 eggs
- ¼ tsp salt
- 2 oz. cheddar cheese
- 1 garlic clove
- ¼ tsp dill

Instructions:

In a bowl, whisk eggs with salt and cheese.

In a frying pan, heat olive oil and pour egg mixture.

Add remaining ingredients and mix well.

Serve when ready.

13. Baked Salmon

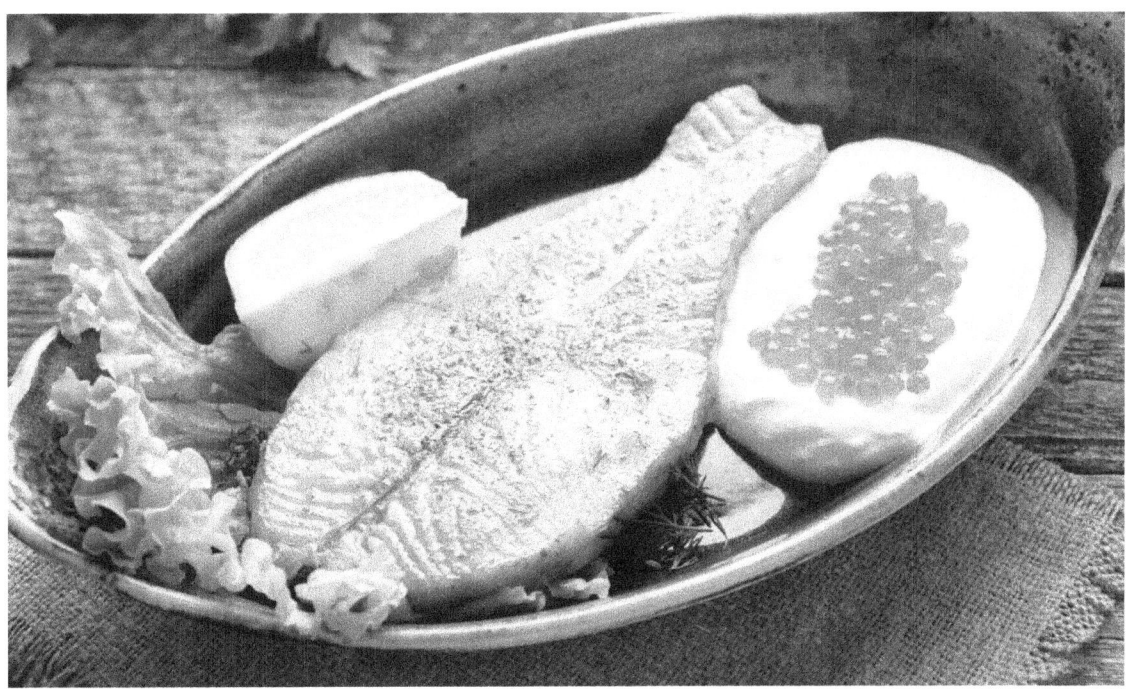

Nourish your body with our Baked Salmon recipe, a lymphedema-friendly delight. Packed with omega-3 fatty acids, this dish promotes inflammation reduction and aids lymphatic system health.

Cooking time: 30 minutes

Servings: 4

Ingredients:

- 4 salmon fillets
- 1 tablespoon butter
- 1 tsp salt
- ¼ tsp pepper
- 1 lemon

Instructions:

Place the salmon on a baking sheet.

Spread melted butter over the salmon.

Sprinkle it with salmon and pepper.

Spread lemon slices over the salmon fillet.

Bake at 400 F for 18-20 minutes.

When ready, remove from the oven and serve.

14. Parmesan Drumsticks

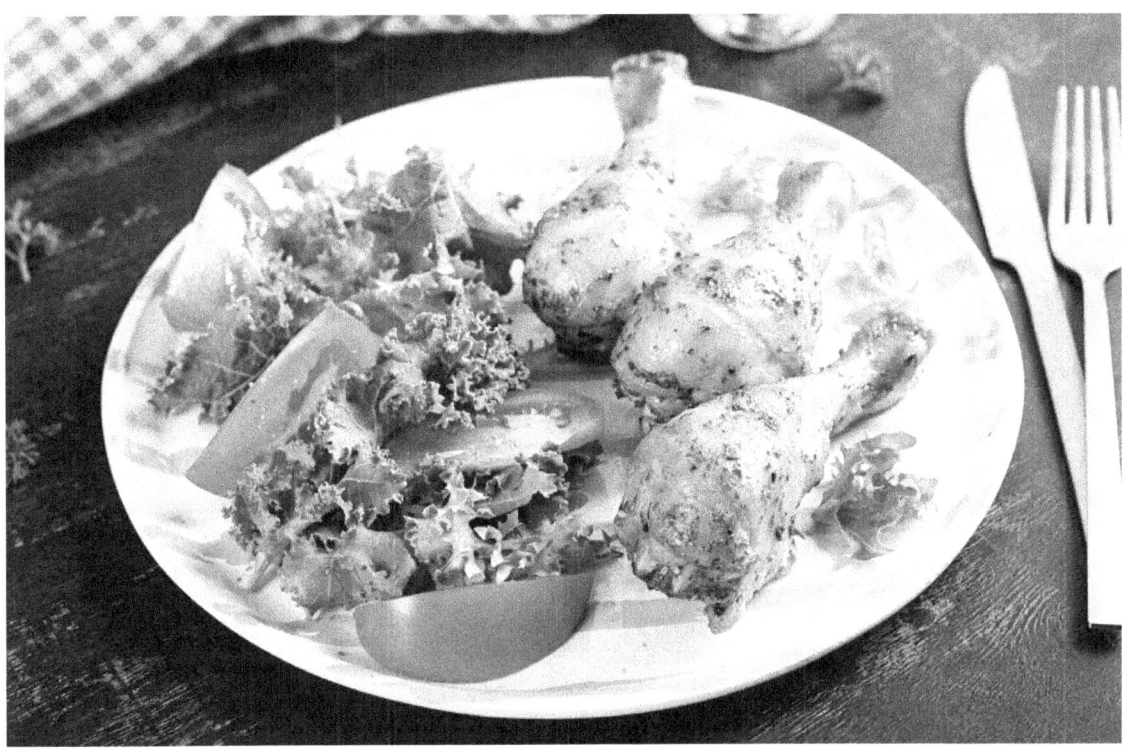

Savoring a delectable solution for lymphedema, Parmesan Drumsticks offer a flavorful twist on a nutritious journey. They are packed with protein and low in sodium and cater to a health-conscious audience.

Cooking time: 50 minutes

Servings: 3

Ingredients:

- 2 eggs
- 2 cups parmesan cheese
- 1 tsp salt
- 1 tsp black pepper
- 12 chicken drumsticks
- 2 tbsp. coconut oil

Instructions:

Preheat the oven to 375 F.

In a bowl, crack eggs, beat them and set aside.

In another bowl, mix cheese, pepper, salt and set aside.

Dip the drumsticks into the egg mixture and coat evenly.

Roll into cheese mixture and place in the baking pan.

Bake for 40-50 minutes, remove and serve.

15. Cauliflower Soup

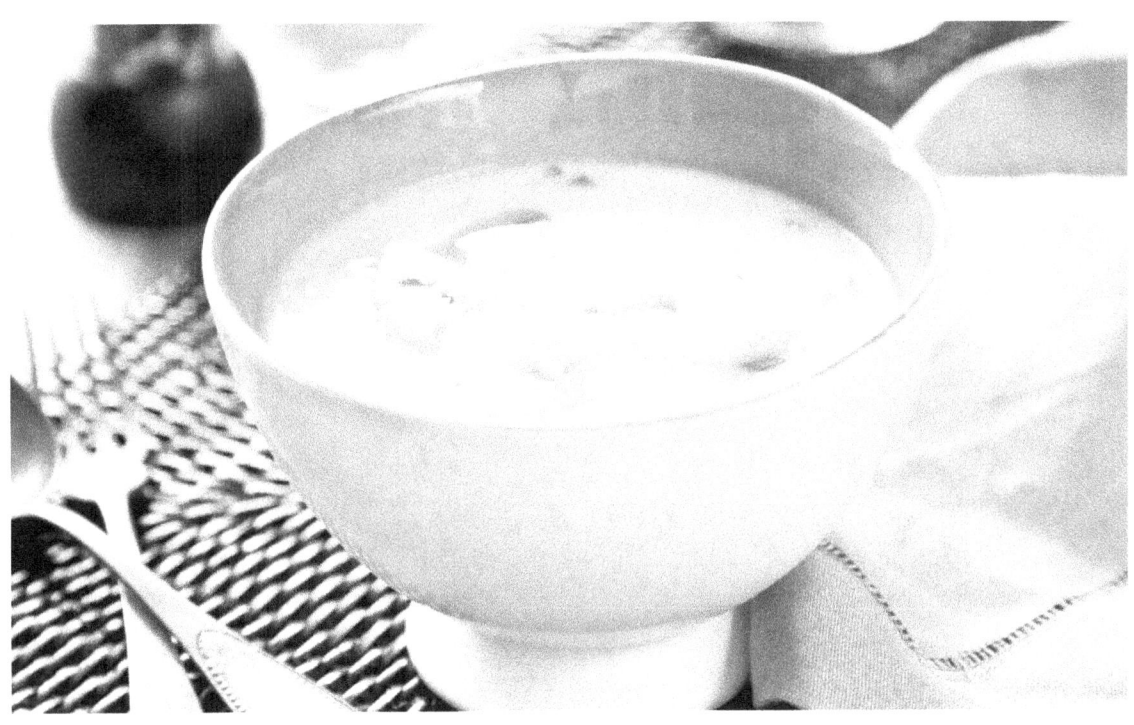

This recipe is a boon for those managing lymphedema, as it supports a balanced diet. Its velvety texture and mild flavor make it suitable for everyone, promoting overall well-being without compromising on taste.

Cooking time: 30 minutes

Servings: 4

Ingredients:

- 1 tablespoon olive oil
- 1 lb. cauliflower
- ¼ red onion
- ½ cup all-purpose flour
- ¼ tsp. salt
- ¼ tsp. pepper
- 1 can vegetable broth
- 1 cup heavy cream

Instructions:

In a saucepan, heat olive oil and sauté cauliflower until tender.

Add remaining ingredients to the saucepan and bring to a boil.

When all the vegetables are tender, transfer to a blender and blend until smooth.

Pour soup into bowls, garnish with parsley and serve.

16. Soy-Free Cup Chicken

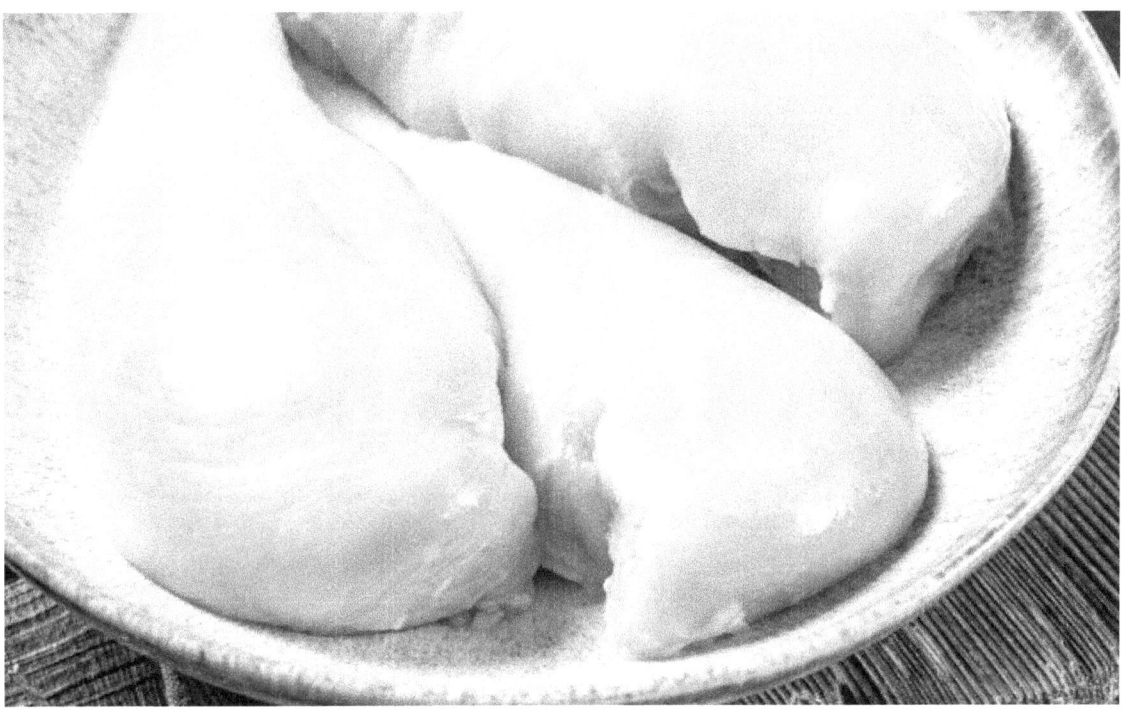

This recipe is not only delicious but also suitable for all, accommodating various dietary preferences. With its balanced ingredients, it promotes lymphatic health and is a tasty addition to your meal repertoire.

Cooking time: 55 minutes

Servings: 6

Ingredients:

- 10 oz. chicken breast
- 3 tbsp. sesame oil
- 3-inch ginger
- 15 garlic cloves
- 1 tsp. black pepper
- 1 pinch ground cloves
- 2 tbsp. coconut aminos
- 1 tbsp. fish sauce
- 1 tbsp. honey
- 1 cup basil leaves

Instructions:

In a skillet, add sesame oil over medium heat.

Add garlic, pepper, ginger, cloves and sauté for 2-3 minutes

Add chicken and cook for 5-10 minutes.

Add honey, fish sauce, coconut aminos and bring to a boil.

Simmer for 12-15 minutes, remove from heat, add basil leaves and serve.

17. Chicken Lettuce Wraps

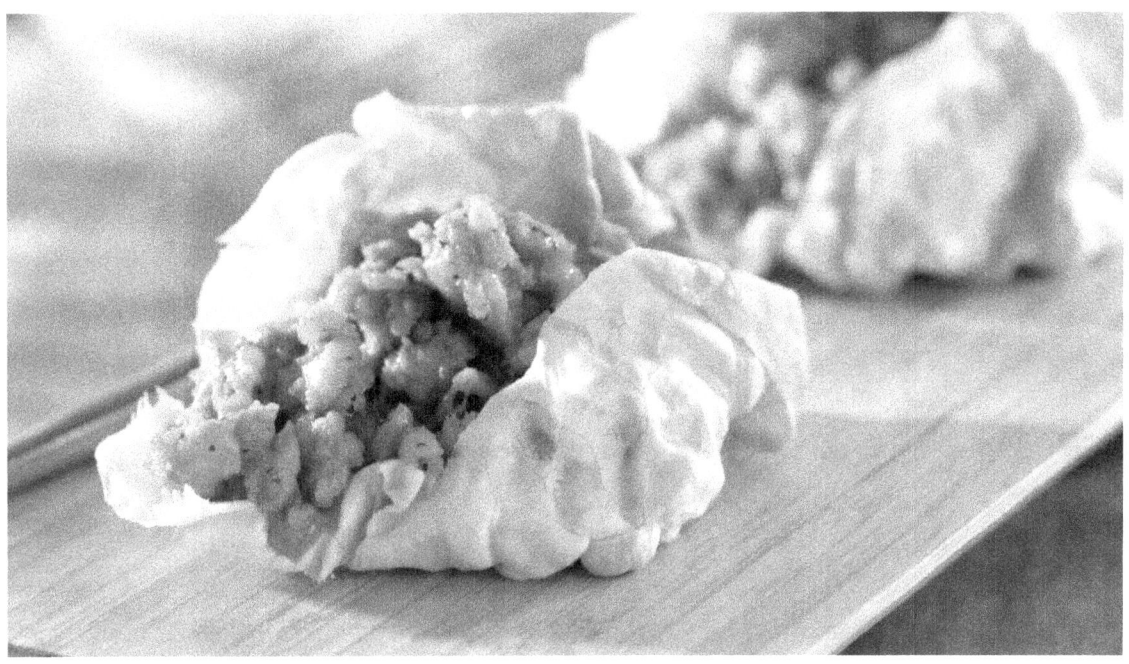

These Chicken Lettuce Wraps offer a health-conscious twist on a classic favorite. Packed with lean protein and fresh vegetables, they're a guilt-free delight suitable for all. The crisp lettuce cups provide a refreshing crunch, while the flavorful chicken filling brings a satisfying taste.

Cooking time: 30 minutes

Servings: 2

Ingredients:

- 2 lbs. ground chicken
- 2 onions
- 3 garlic cloves
- 1 yellow squash
- 1 bell pepper
- 1 bunch basil
- ½ tsp salt
- 1 cup Italian dressing
- 1 head romaine lettuce

Instructions:

Cook ground chicken until tender with garlic, pepper, basil, onions, and squash.

Serve the squash with lettuce leaves and Italian dressing.

18. French Pot Roast

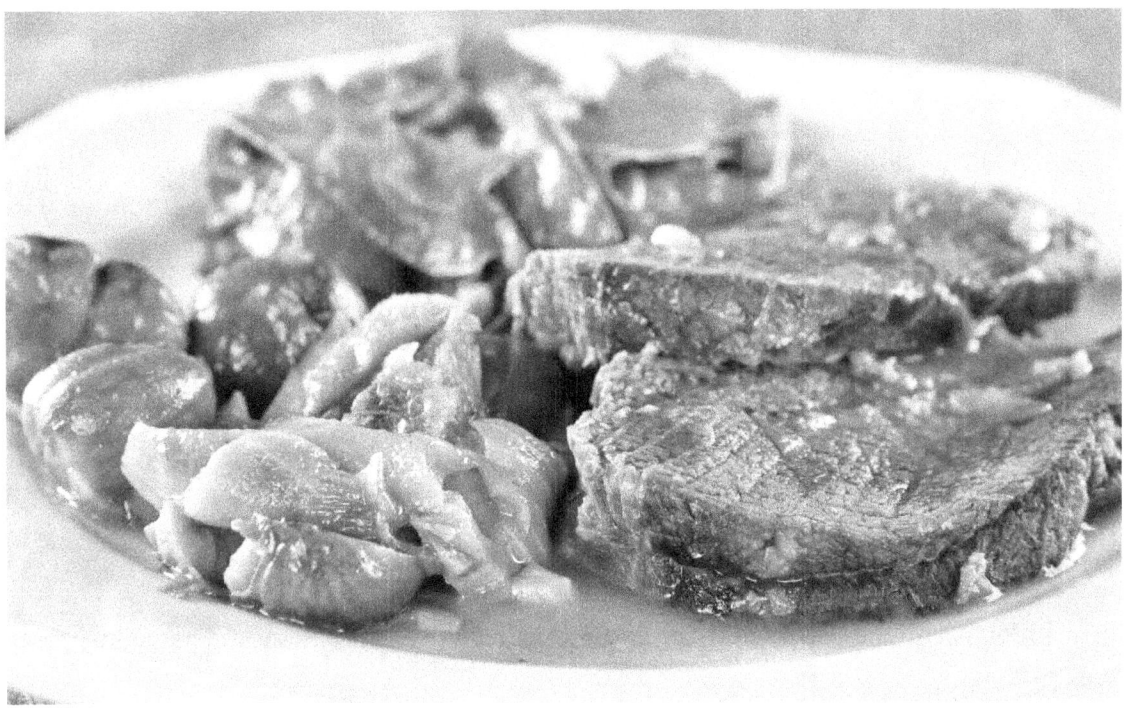

This is a hearty and comforting dish that's a perfect choice for those seeking a wholesome and satisfying meal. Packed with tender, slow-cooked meat and a medley of vegetables, this recipe not only delights the taste buds but also provides essential nutrients.

Cooking time: 7 hours 10 minutes

Servings: 4

Ingredients:

- 1 tbsp. butter
- 2 lbs. beef roast
- 1 onion
- 6 cloves garlic
- 3 slices bacon
- ¼ cup red wine
- ½ tsp. rosemary
- ¼ tsp. dried thyme
- Pinch of salt

Instructions:

In a skillet, heat butter, add beef roast and brown on all sides, remove and place in a crock pot.

Sauté onions, bacon, garlic and move to a crock pot.

Add onion, seasoning and cook on low for 6-7 hours.

19. Tomatoes & Ham Pizza

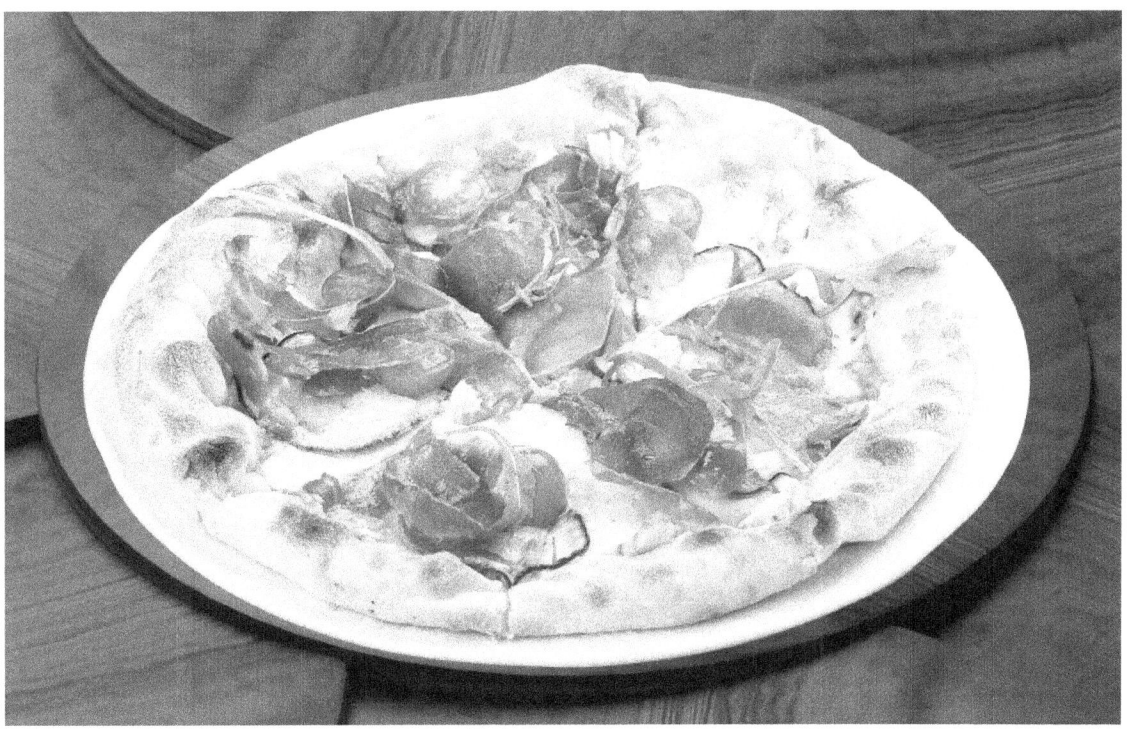

Elevate your taste buds with our Tomatoes & Ham Pizza, a lymphedema-friendly delight. Packed with juicy tomatoes and lean ham, it's a delicious, guilt-free option for everyone. The balanced blend of flavors not only satisfies cravings but also caters to those mindful of lymphedema concerns.

Cooking time: 25 minutes

Servings: 8

Ingredients:

- 1 pizza crust
- ½ cup tomato sauce
- ¼ black pepper
- 1 cup pepperoni slices
- 1 cup tomatoes
- 6-8 ham slices
- 1 cup mozzarella cheese
- 1 cup olives

Instructions:

Spread tomato sauce on the pizza crust.

Place all the toppings on the pizza crust.

Bake the pizza at 425 F for 12-15 minutes.

When ready, remove pizza from the oven and serve.

20. Chicken Curry Soup

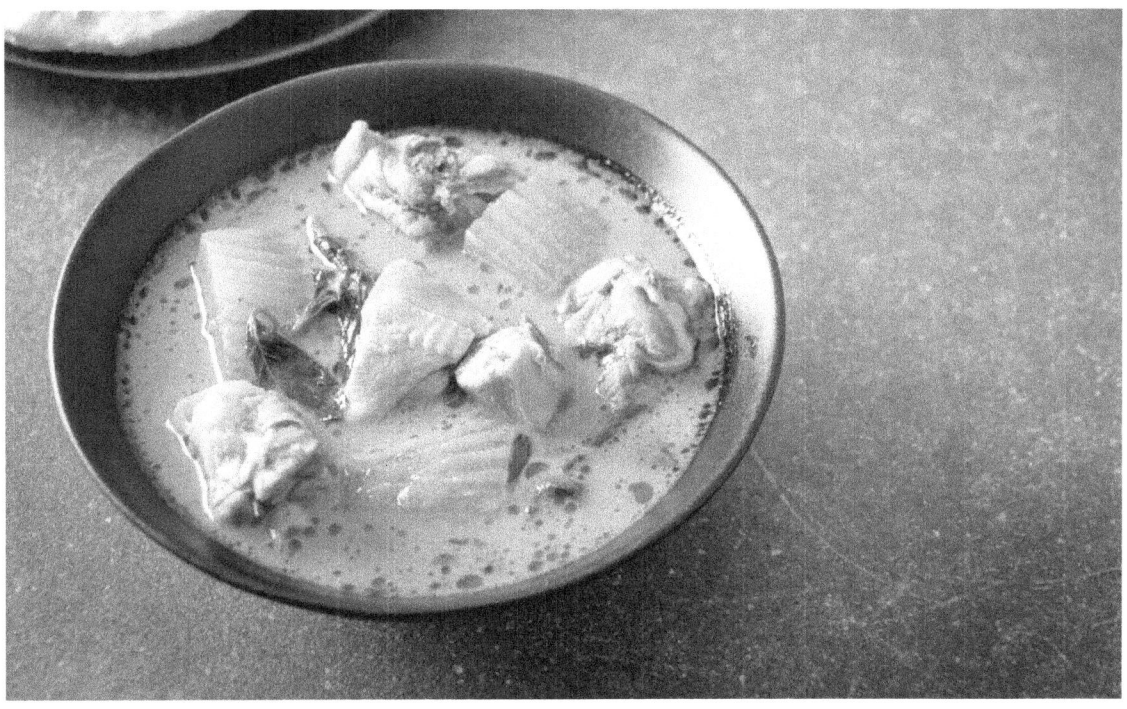

This Chicken Curry Soup is a nutritious delight that's perfect for everyone. Packed with lean protein and anti-inflammatory spices, it's a comforting and healthy choice.

Cooking time: 100 minutes

Servings: 12

Ingredients:

- 1 chicken
- coconut oil
- 1 onion
- 3 cups rhubarb
- 3 cloves garlic
- 1-inch ginger
- 1 tbsp. coriander
- 10 vegetables

Instructions:

In a pot, add giblets, chicken, and cover with water.

Bring to boil and cook for 60 minutes, heat a cast iron pan over medium heat.

Add coconut oil, onion, rhubarb and sauté for 10-12 minutes.

Add ginger, spices, garlic, stir in and sauté for 2-3 minutes.

Remove chicken from the pot and place on a plate.

Add rhubarb mixture and vegetables into the soup and simmer for 25-30 minutes.

Add chicken back, stir to combine and serve.

Chapter 3: Dessert Recipes

21. Chocolate Tart

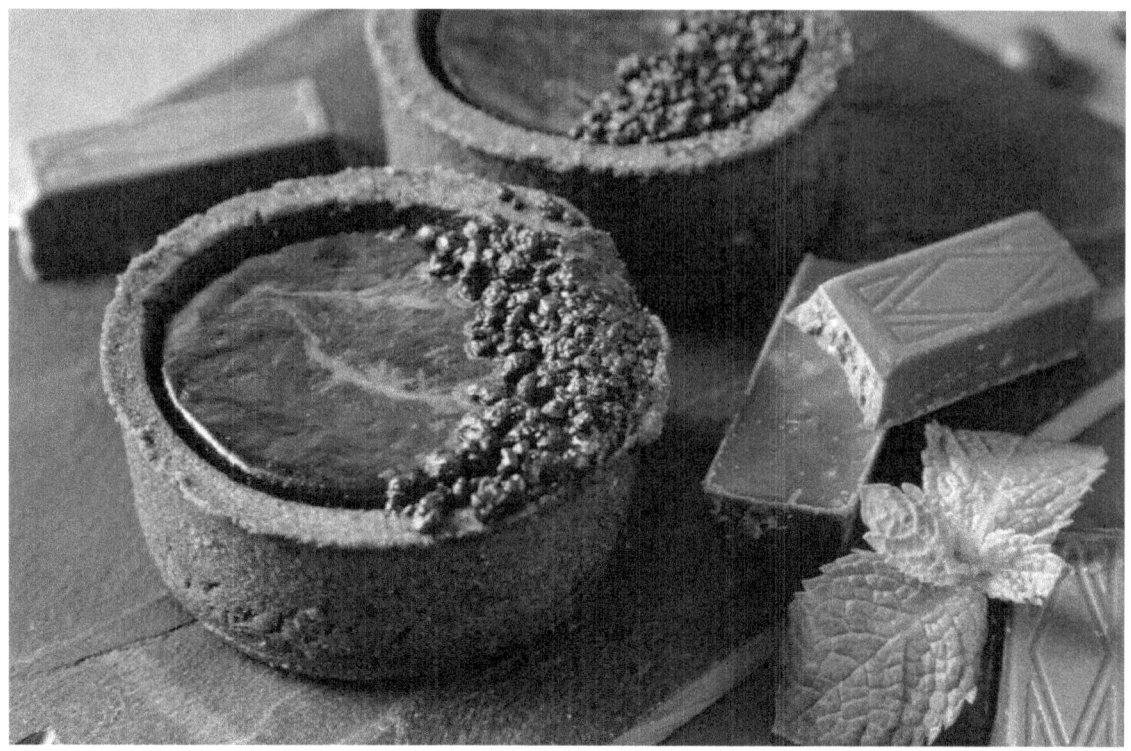

Indulging in a rich, velvety Chocolate Tart doesn't have to be a guilty pleasure anymore. This delectable treat boasts a gluten-free almond crust and a creamy, dairy-free chocolate filling that's gentle on your lymphatic system.

Cooking time: 50 minutes

Servings: 6

Ingredients:

- Pastry sheets
- 1 tsp vanilla extract
- ½ lb. caramel
- ½ lb. black chocolate
- 4-5 tablespoons butter
- 3 eggs
- ¼ lb. brown sugar

Instructions:

Preheat the oven to 400 F, unfold pastry sheets and place them on a baking sheet.

Toss all ingredients together and mix well.

Spread mixture in a single layer on the pastry sheets.

Before baking, decorate with your desired fruits.

Bake at 400 F for 22-25 minutes or until golden brown.

22. Gingerbread Biscuits

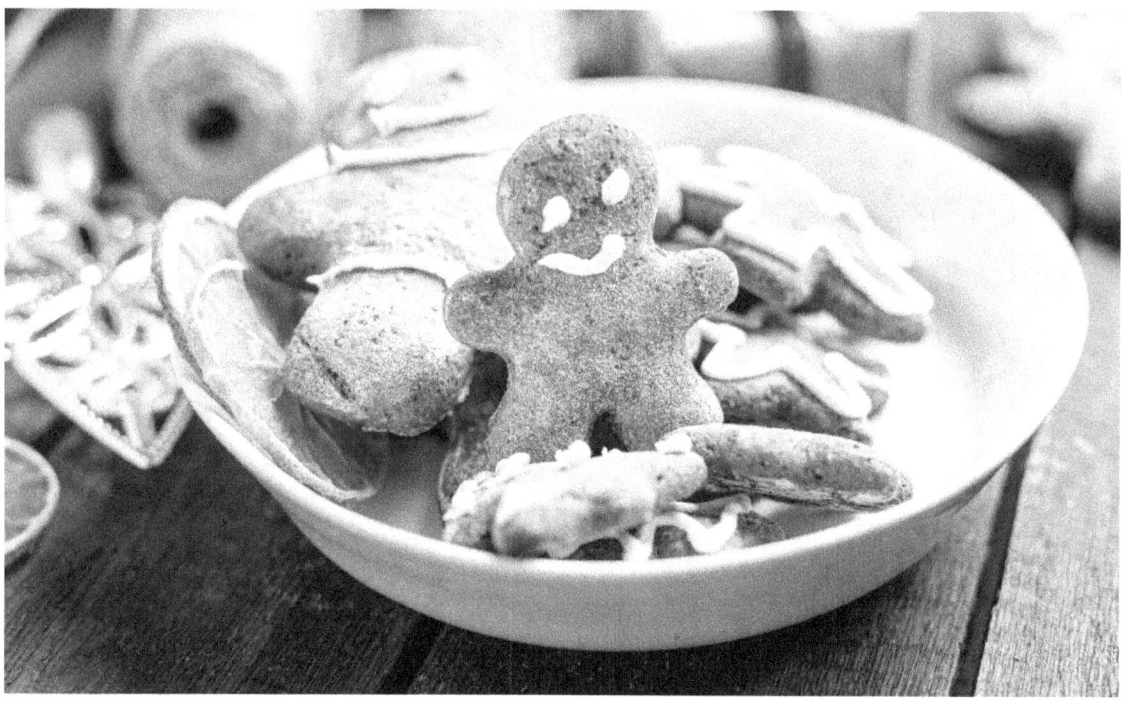

These Gingerbread Biscuits are a delightful blend of sweet and spicy, perfect for anyone looking to enjoy a guilt-free treat. Packed with the goodness of ginger, these biscuits not only satisfy your taste buds but also offer potential anti-inflammatory benefits.

Cooking time: 40 minutes

Servings: 4

Ingredients:

- 2 oz. butter
- 1 cup self-raising flour
- ½ tsp salt
- 3 tablespoons ginger
- ½ cup milk
- 1 egg beaten
- 1 tablespoon vanilla extract
- ½ cup golden syrup
- ½ cup maple syrup
- ½ cup honey

Instructions:

Preheat the oven to 300 F.

In a pan, melt honey, butter, syrup and set aside.

White syrup mixture is cooling, grate the ginger and add to the syrup mixture.

Add flour, salt, milk, egg and vanilla extract.

Form small cookies and bake for 15-18 minutes at 300 F.

Remove and serve.

23. Grapefruit Pie

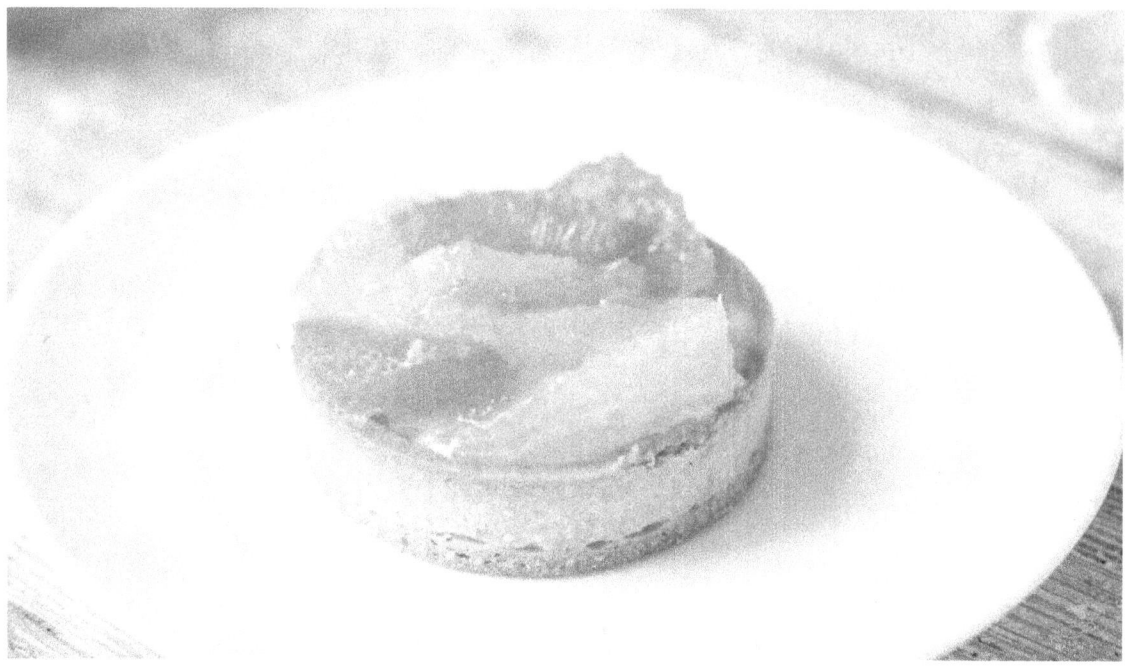

Treat your taste buds to a zesty delight with our Grapefruit Pie recipe! Packed with tangy grapefruit goodness, this dessert offers a refreshing twist on classic pie.

Cooking time: 50 minutes

Servings: 8

Ingredients:

- Pastry sheets
- 2 cups grapefruit
- 1 cup brown sugar
- ¼ cup flour
- 5-6 egg yolks
- 5 oz. butter

Instructions:

Line a pie plate or pie form with pastry and cover the edges of the plate depending on your preference.

In a bowl, combine all pie ingredients together and mix well.

Pour the mixture over the pastry.

Bake at 400-425 F for 25-30 minutes or until golden brown.

When ready, remove from the oven and let it rest for 15 minutes.

24. Cucumber Chips

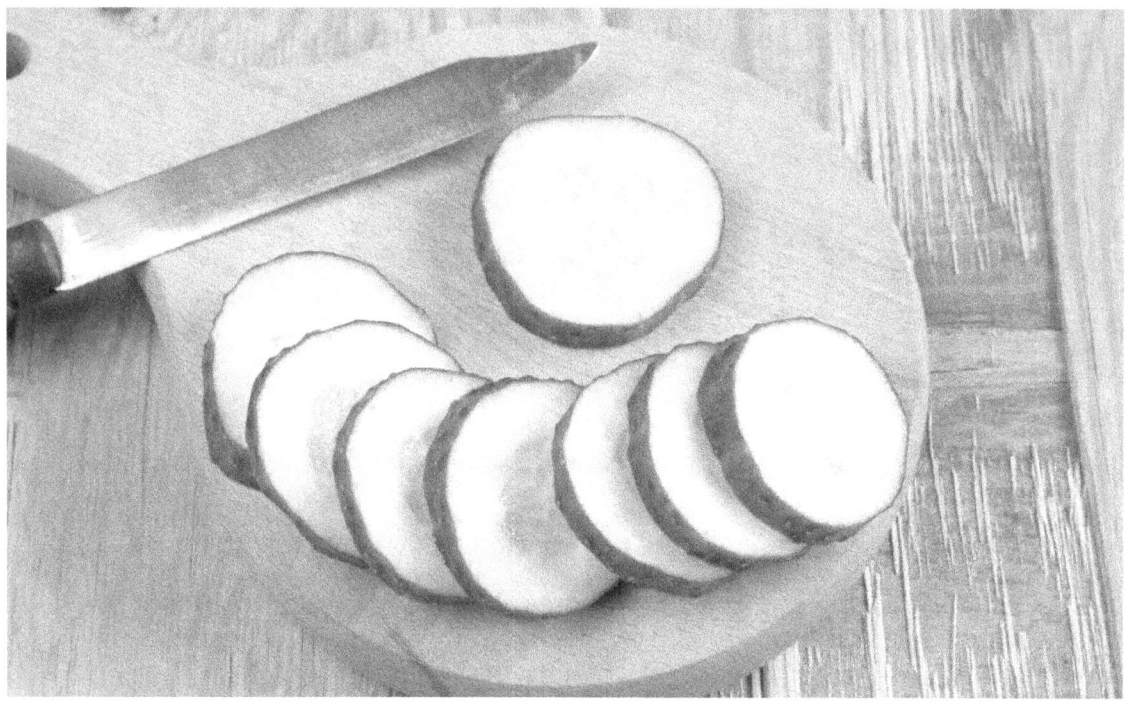

Crispy and refreshing, Cucumber Chips are a guilt-free snack that's as good for your taste buds as it is for your health. Packed with hydrating cucumbers, they're a low-calorie alternative to traditional chips. Whether you're watching your waistline or simply seeking a tasty, crunchy treat, these chips are suitable for all.

Cooking time: 30 minutes

Servings: 2

Ingredients:

- 1 lb. cucumber
- 1 tablespoon olive oil
- 1 tablespoon parmesan cheese
- 1 tsp garlic powder
- 1 tsp seasoning

Instructions:

Preheat the oven to 425 F

In a bowl, toss everything with olive oil and seasoning

Spread everything onto a prepared baking sheet.

Bake for 8-10 minutes or until crisp.

When ready, remove from the oven and serve.

25. Sweet Potato Fries

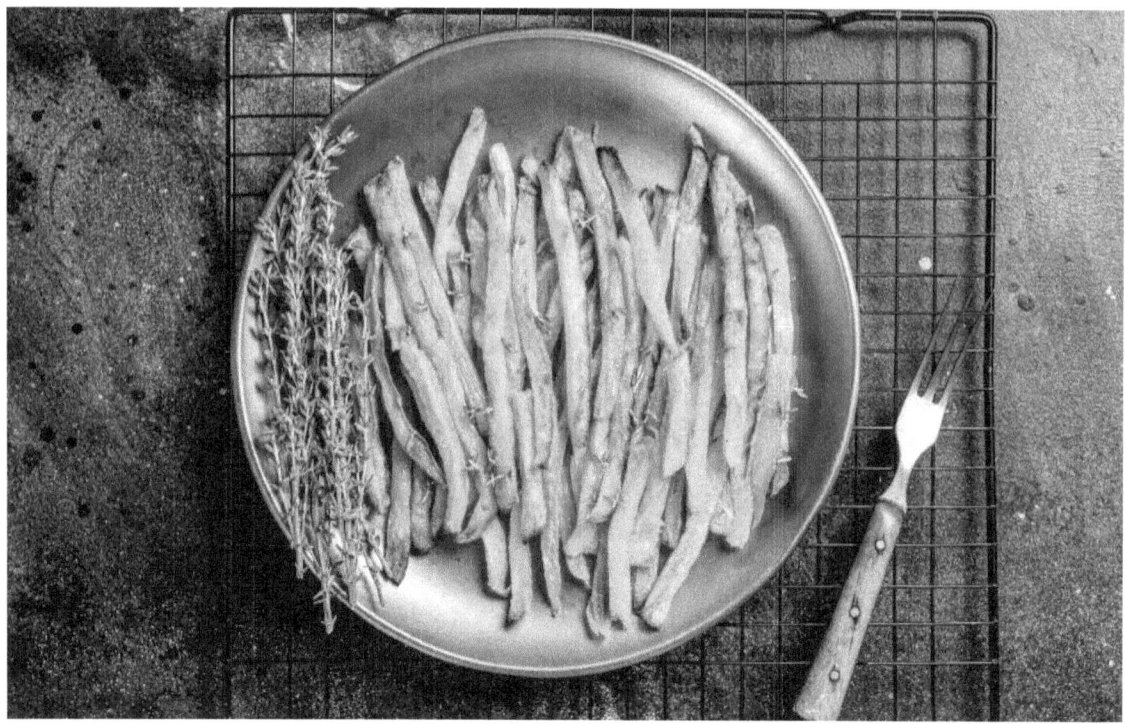

These Sweet Potato Fries are a delicious and nutritious treat that everyone can enjoy. Packed with vitamins and fiber, they're a guilt-free snack or side dish.

Cooking time: 40 minutes

Servings: 2

Ingredients:

- 1 lb. sweet potatoes
- ¼ tsp. garlic powder
- ¼ tsp. paprika
- ¼ tsp. salt
- ½ cup parmesan

Instructions:

Cut potatoes into thick wedges.

Place them on a baking sheet.

Sprinkle with seasoning and toss to coat.

Roast at 400 F for 25-30 minutes or until golden.

When ready, remove from the oven and serve with parmesan cheese.

26. Simple Pizza

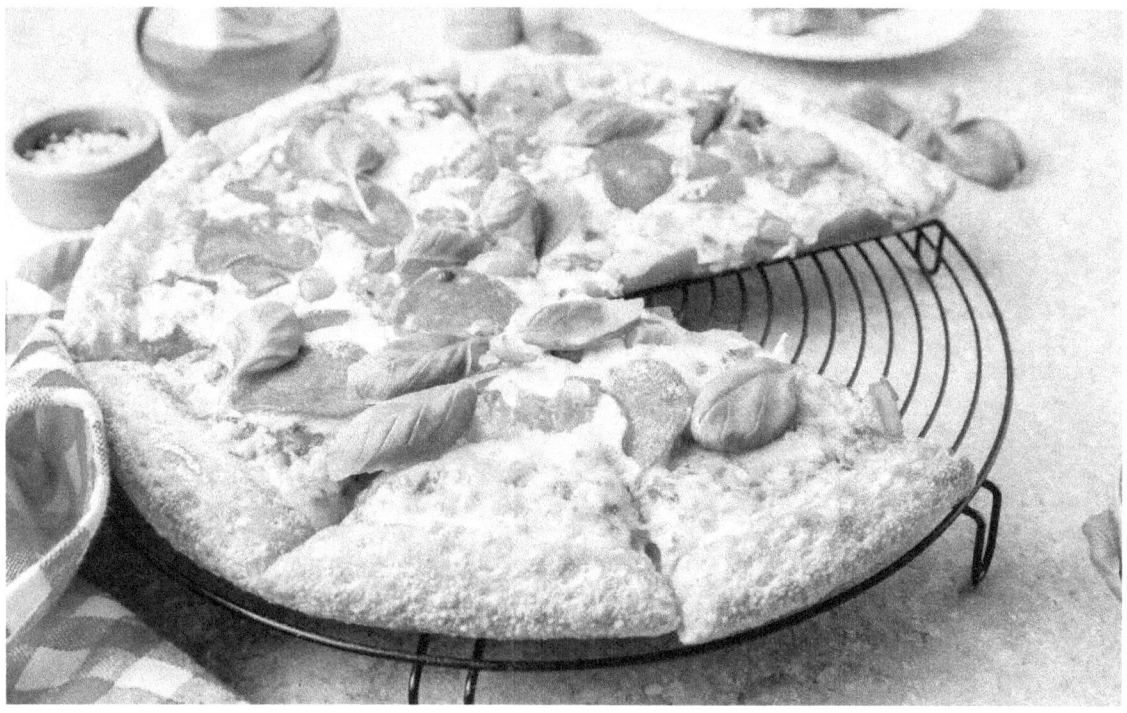

Packed with fresh veggies, lean protein, and a whole wheat crust, it's a delicious way to satisfy your pizza cravings without compromising your health.

Cooking time: 25 minutes

Servings: 6

Ingredients:

- 1 pizza crust
- ½ cup tomato sauce
- ¼ black pepper
- 1 cup pepperoni slices
- 1 cup mozzarella cheese
- 1 cup olives

Instructions:

Spread tomato sauce on the pizza crust.

Place all the toppings on the pizza crust.

Bake the pizza at 425 F for 12-15 minutes.

When ready, remove pizza from the oven and serve.

27. Roasted Chickpeas

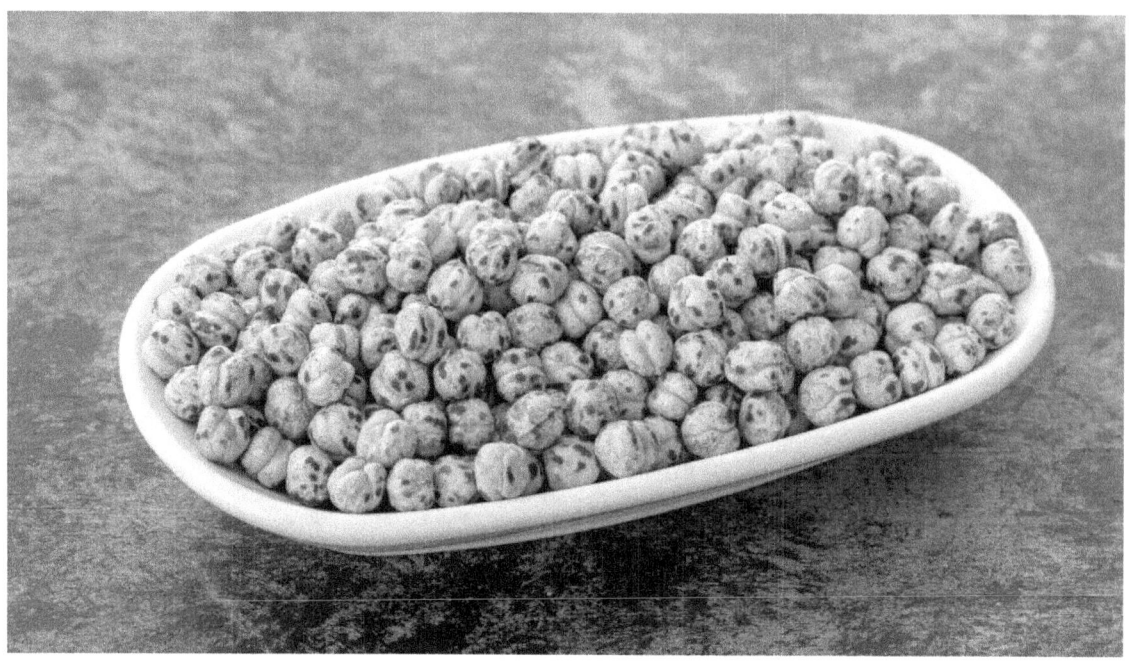

Roasted Chickpeas: a crunchy, savory snack that's as nutritious as it is delicious. These little powerhouses are rich in protein and fiber, making them a satisfying and healthy option for all snack lovers. Say goodbye to guilt and hello to flavor-packed, guilt-free munching!

Cooking time: 40 minutes

Servings: 4

Ingredients:

- 2 cups chickpeas
- 2 tsp olive oil
- 1 tsp salt
- ¼ tsp smoked paprika
- ¼ tsp garlic powder

Instructions:

Place the chickpeas on a baking sheet.

Sprinkle the seasoning over the chickpeas.

Drizzle olive oil and toss to coat.

Bake at 400 F for 28-30 minutes or until they are crunchy.

When ready, remove from the oven and serve.

28. Caramel Popcorn

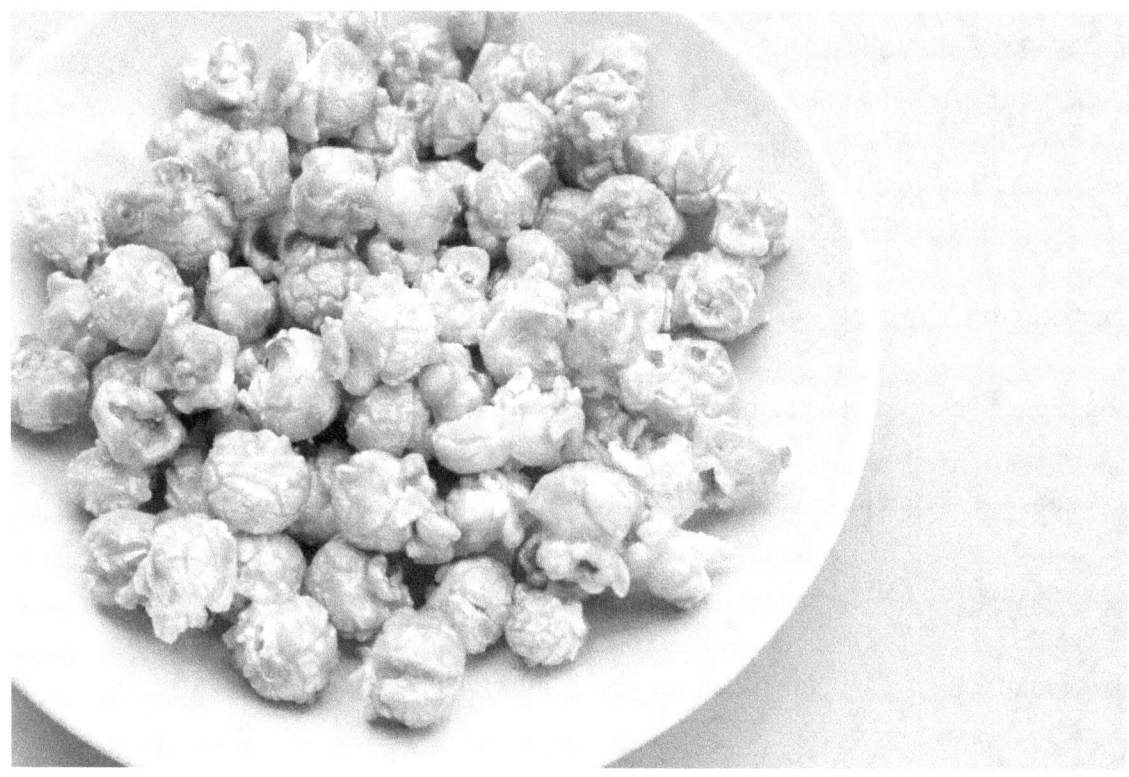

This recipe offers the perfect balance of buttery caramel and crunchy popcorn. It's a crowd-pleaser, ideal for movie nights or sharing with friends. The gooey caramel coating adds a touch of indulgence to this classic recipe.

Cooking time: 30 minutes

Servings: 4

Ingredients:

- 1 tablespoon olive oil
- 4 tablespoons popcorn kernels

Caramel Sauce:

- 1 tablespoon butter
- 1 tablespoon brown sugar
- 1 tablespoon golden syrup

Instructions:

In a saucepan, pour olive oil and popcorn kernels over medium heat and cover.

Shake the saucepan to distribute evenly.

In another saucepan, melt the caramel sauce ingredients.

Remove from heat and pour over your popcorn.

29. Chocolate Muffins

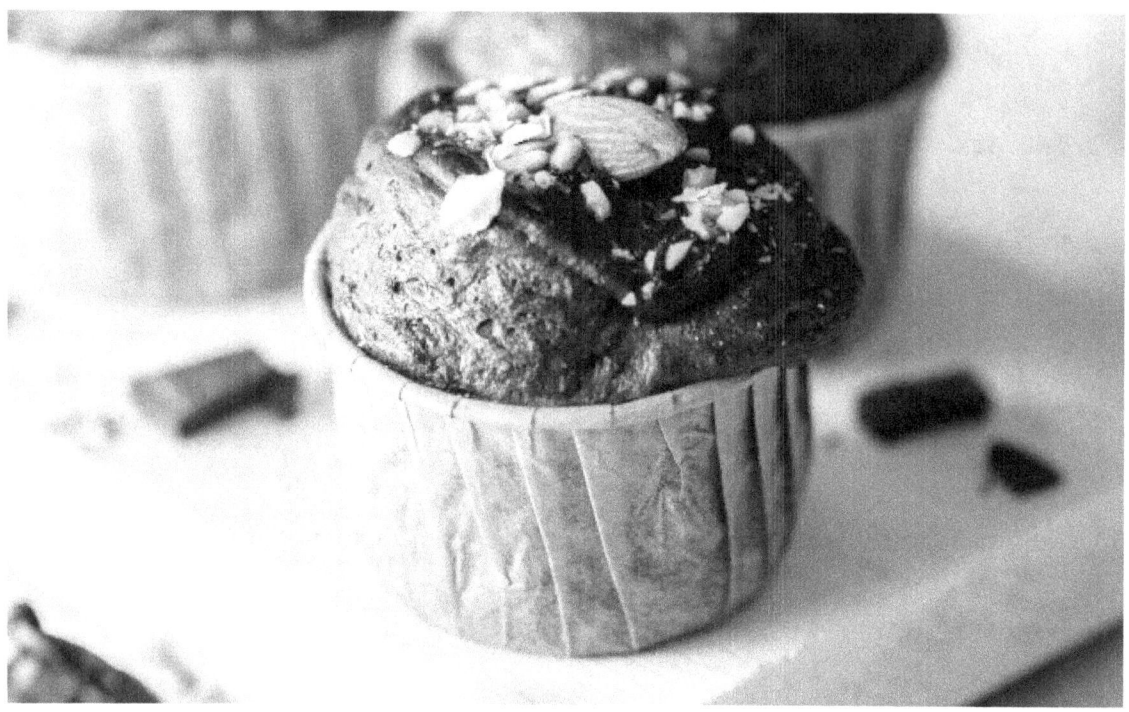

These Chocolate Muffins aren't just a tasty treat; they're a guilt-free delight for everyone! Packed with rich cocoa flavor, they're secretly low in sugar and high in fiber, making them a perfect choice for those with dietary restrictions.

Cooking time: 30 minutes

Servings: 8

Ingredients:

- 2 eggs
- 1 tablespoon olive oil
- 1 cup milk
- 2 cups whole wheat flour
- 1 tsp baking soda
- ¼ tsp baking soda
- 1 tsp cinnamon
- 1 cup chocolate chips

Instructions:

In a bowl, combine all dry ingredients.

In another bowl, combine all dry ingredients.

Combine wet and dry ingredients together.

Pour mixture into 8-12 prepared muffin cups, fill 2/3 of the cups.

Bake for 18-20 minutes at 375 F.

When ready, remove from the oven and serve.

30. Cheese Cake

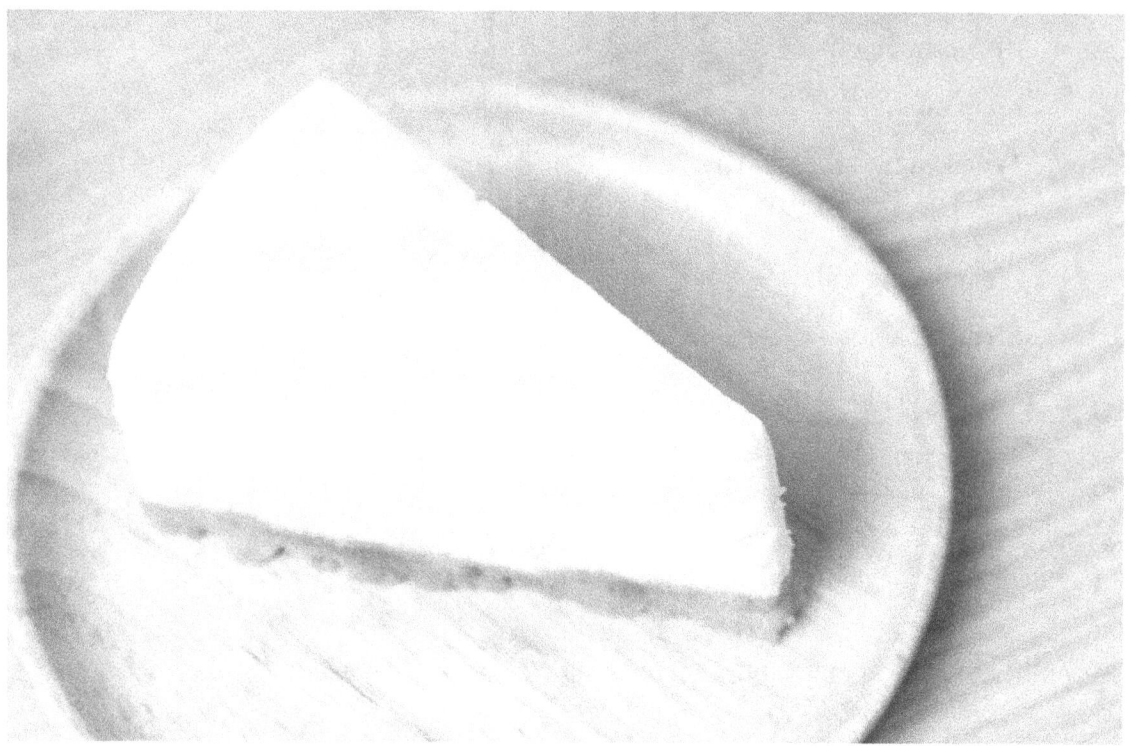

This delightful cheesecake recipe offers a guilt-free twist on a classic favorite. With a creamy, rich texture and a hint of sweetness, it's a treat that won't leave you feeling heavy. What's even better? It's suitable for all, including those with dietary restrictions, making it a versatile and satisfying dessert option.

Cooking time: 40 minutes

Servings: 4

Ingredients:

- ½ lb. gingernut biscuits
- ½ lb. blueberries
- 1 tsp vanilla extract
- 1 tsp acid
- ¼ lb. butter
- ¼ lb. caster sugar
- 2 tablespoons arrowroot
- ¼ lb. full-fat Philadelphia
- 2 eggs

Instructions:

Preheat the oven to 350 F.

In a bowl, mix butter and biscuits and press into the base of the tin.

Bake for 10-12 minutes.

In a saucepan, cook blueberries with sugar and milk for 10-12 minutes.

Take off heat, add citric acid and vanilla.

Bake for 40 minutes, remove and let it chill.

Chapter 4: Salad Recipes

31. Sardines Salad

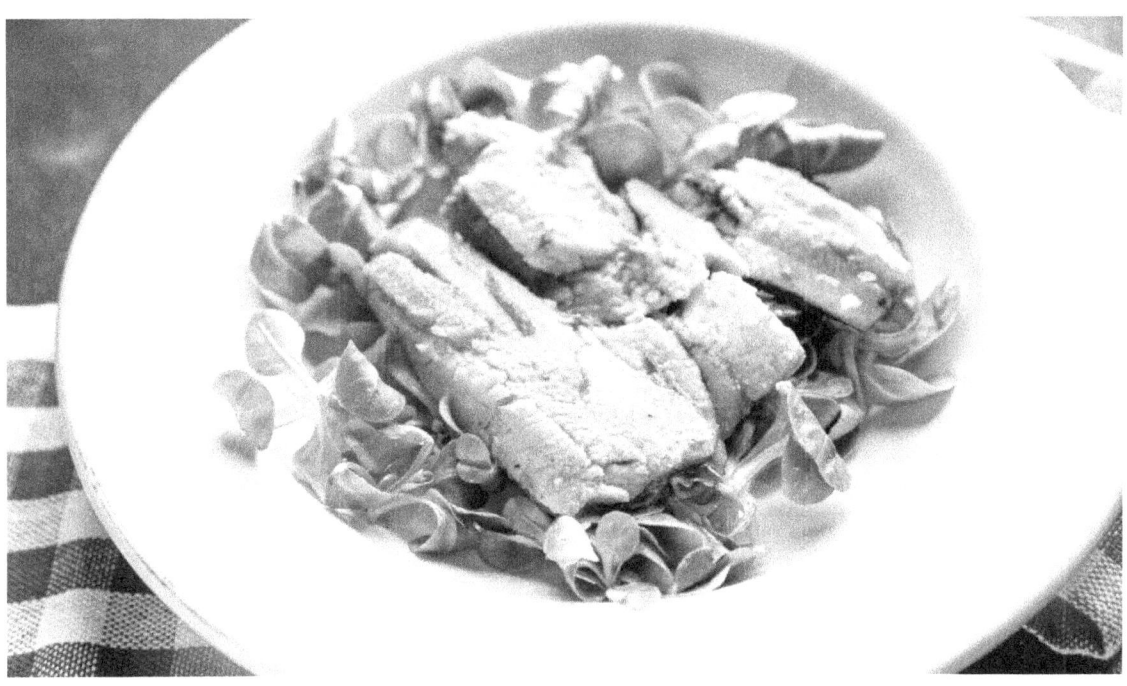

Sardines salad is a nutritious and easy-to-make dish that packs a punch of flavor and health benefits. Packed with omega-3 fatty acids, protein, and essential minerals, it supports heart and brain health.

Cooking time: 10 minutes

Servings: 1

Ingredients:

- 1 can sardines
- ¼ lb. salad greens
- 1 tablespoon olive oil
- 1 tablespoon olive oil
- Pinch of salt

Instructions:

In a bowl, combine all ingredients together and mix well.

Serve with dressing.

32. Tomato Garlic Salad

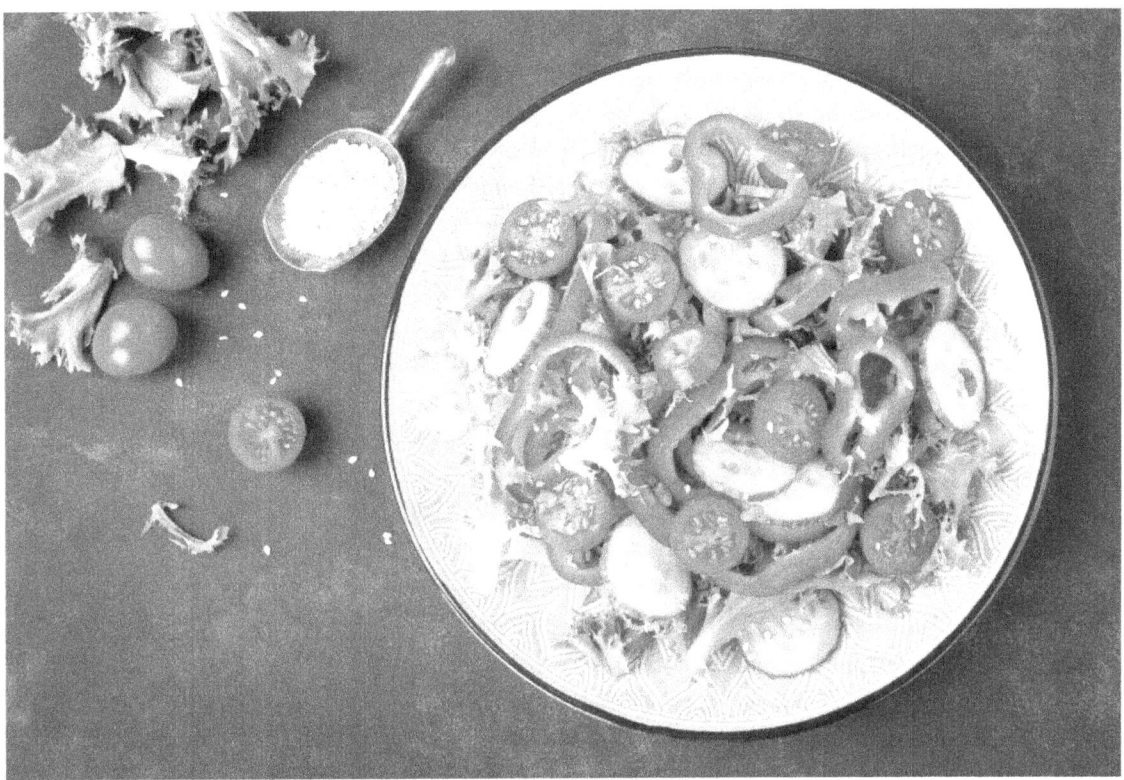

This salad not only tantalizes your taste buds but also boasts numerous health benefits, thanks to the antioxidants in tomatoes and the immune-boosting properties of garlic. It's a delightful, wholesome addition to any meal.

Cooking time: 10 minutes

Servings: 1

Ingredients:

- ¼ cucumber
- ¼ onion
- 1 tomato
- 2 garlic cloves
- 1 tablespoon olive oil
- ½ tsp salt
- 1 basil leaf

Instructions:

In a bowl, combine all ingredients together and mix well.

Serve with dressing.

33. Tuna and Tomatoes Salad

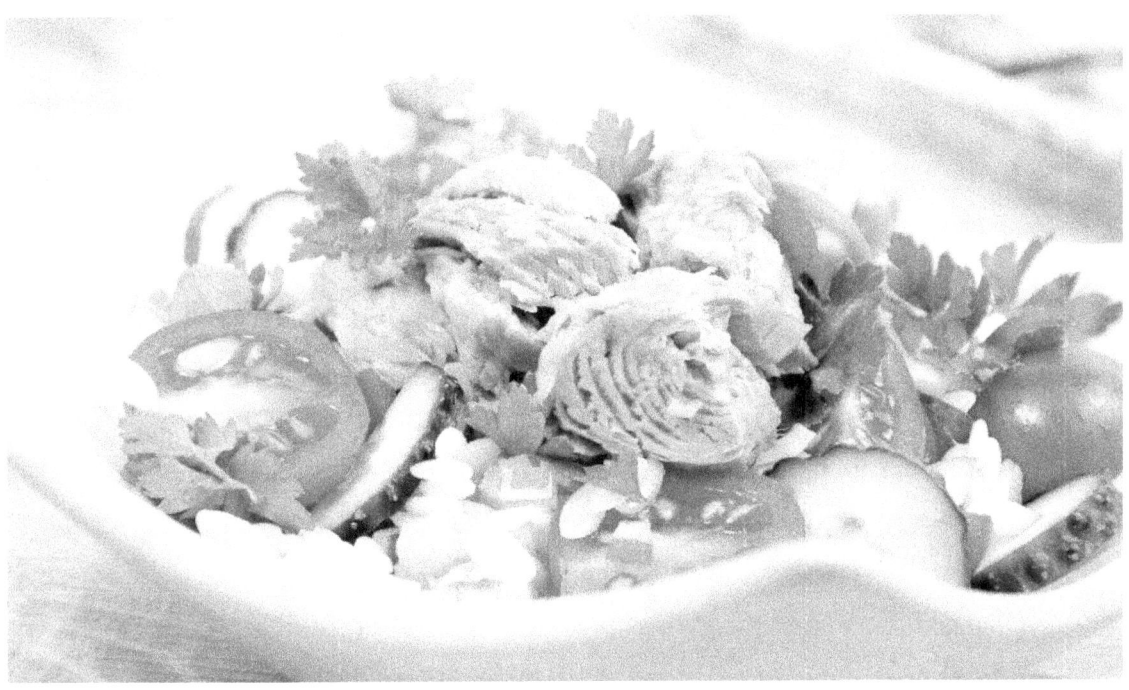

Tuna and tomatoes salad is a delightful, protein-packed dish that's both delicious and nutritious. Succulent chunks of tuna blend perfectly with juicy, ripe tomatoes, creating a medley of flavors and textures.

Cooking time: 10 minutes

Servings: 1

Ingredients:

- 2 tomatoes
- 1 10 oz. can tuna
- ¼ cup onion
- ¼ tsp cumin
- Pinch of salt
- 2 tbsp Lemon juice

Instructions:

In a bowl, combine all ingredients together and mix well.

Serve with dressing.

34. Peach Salad

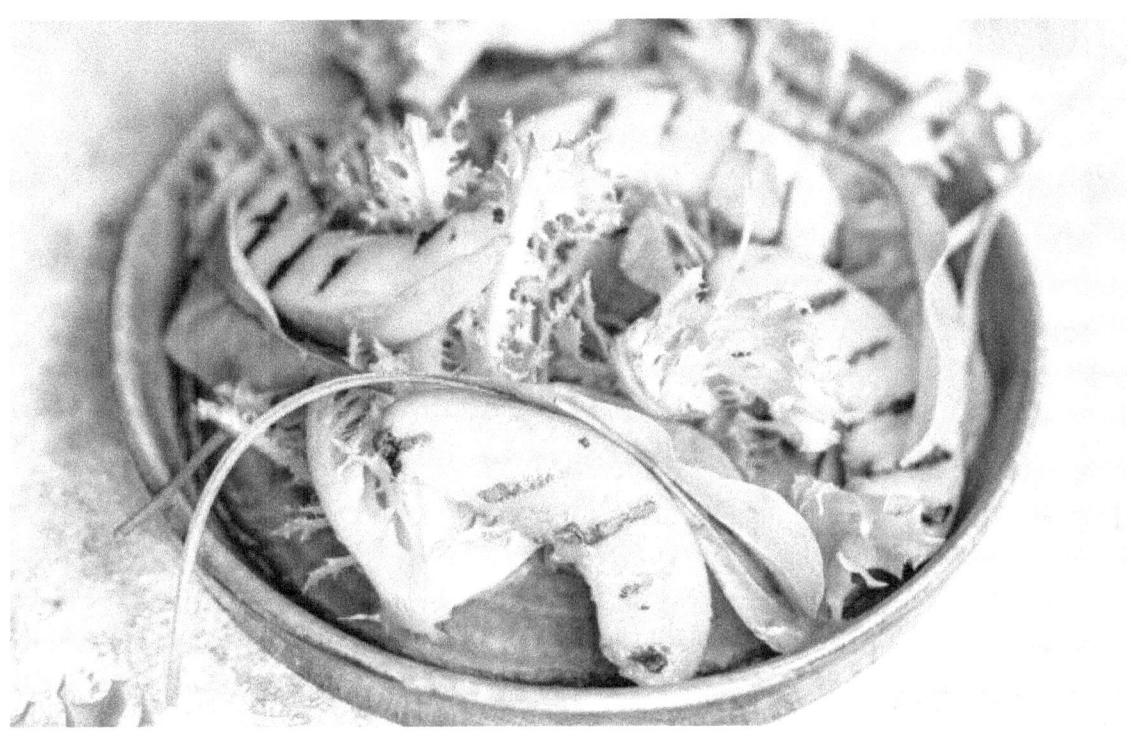

Peach salad is a delightful summer dish that combines the natural sweetness of ripe peaches with a medley of fresh greens. This refreshing salad offers a burst of flavor and nutrition, featuring vitamins, fiber, and antioxidants.

Cooking time: 40 minutes

Servings: 4

Ingredients:

- 1 peach
- 1 handful of pecans
- 1 handful arugula
- 1 handful spinach
- ¼ cup cherry
- 1 tablespoon olive oil
- 1 tablespoon balsamic vinegar

Instructions:

In a bowl, combine all ingredients together and mix well.

Serve with dressing.

35. Watermelon and Lime Salad

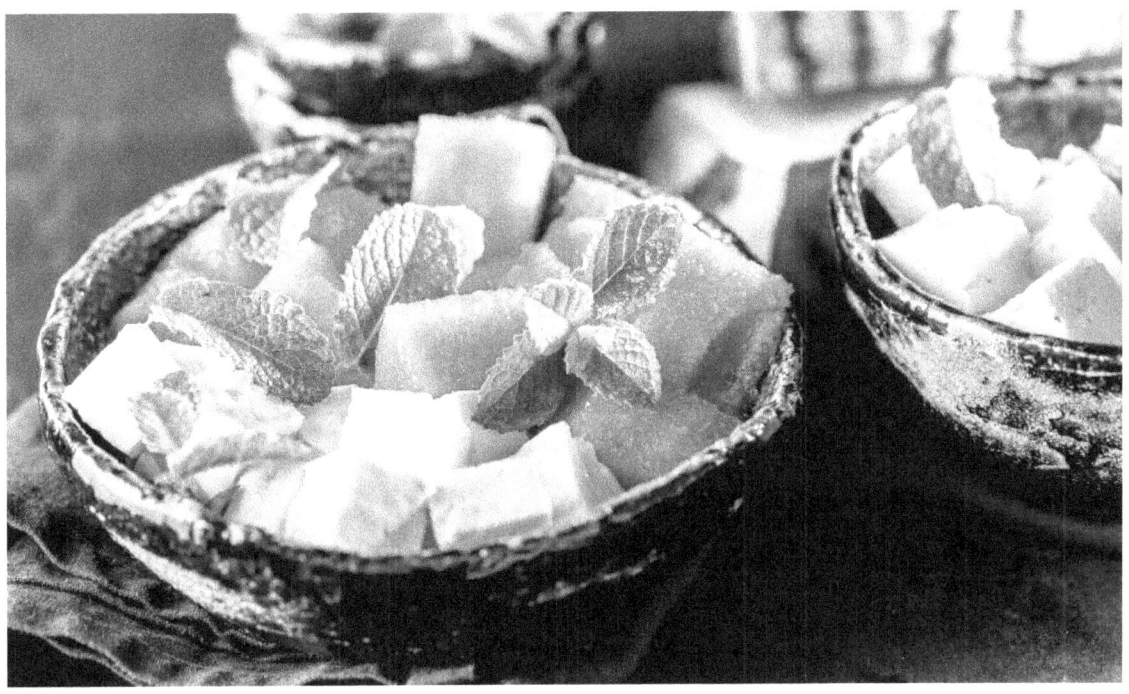

Watermelon and lime salad is the ultimate summer sensation! Crisp, juicy watermelon chunks meet zesty lime in a refreshing explosion of flavors. This salad is not only a delicious treat but also incredibly hydrating, thanks to watermelon's high water content.

Cooking time: 10 minutes

Servings: 4

Ingredients:

- ½ cup onion
- ½ cup lime juice
- 3 cups watermelon
- ½ cup cheddar cheese
- ¼ tsp pepper
- ½ cup cilantro

Instructions:

Soak the onion in the lime juice.

Combine all ingredients into a bowl.

Serve when ready.

36. Paleo Chicken Salad

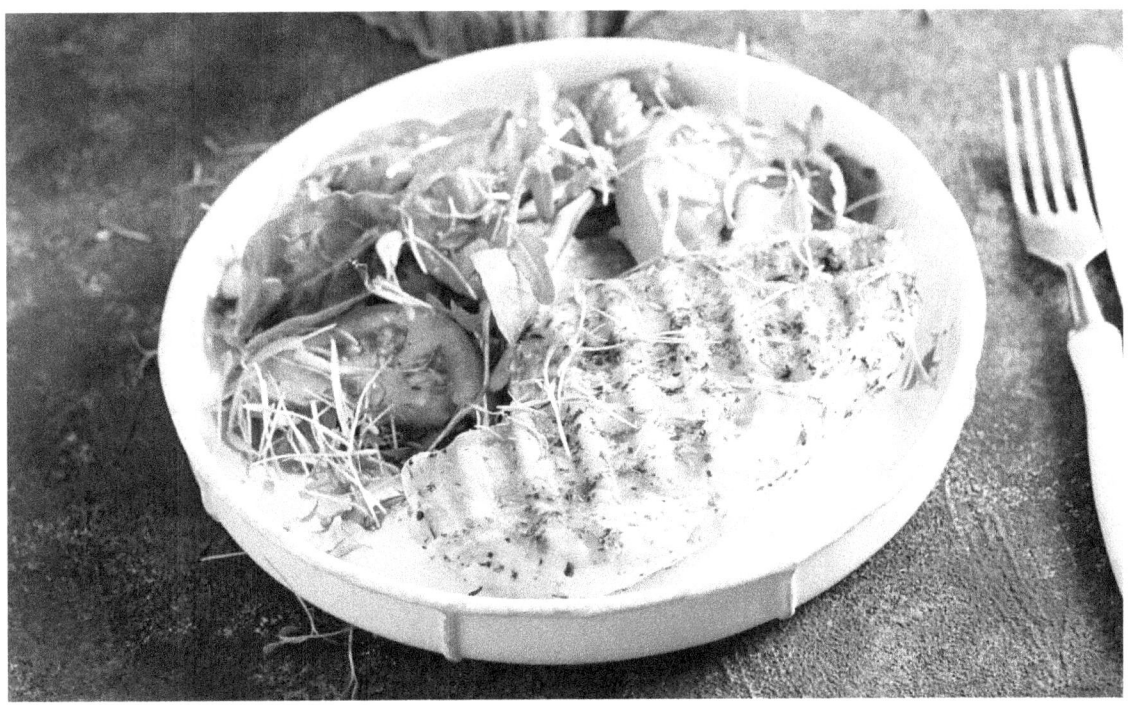

Paleo chicken salad is a wholesome, protein-packed dish that caters to a primal, clean-eating lifestyle. Tender, grilled chicken breast meets a colorful array of fresh vegetables and a flavorful vinaigrette dressing.

Cooking time: 10 minutes

Servings: 1

Ingredients:

- 1 cooked chicken breast
- 2 pieces romaine lettuce
- 1 bell pepper
- 1 carrot
- ¼ red cabbage
- 2 green onions
- Salad dressing

Instructions:

In a bowl, combine all ingredients together and mix well.

Serve with dressing.

37. Arugula Salad

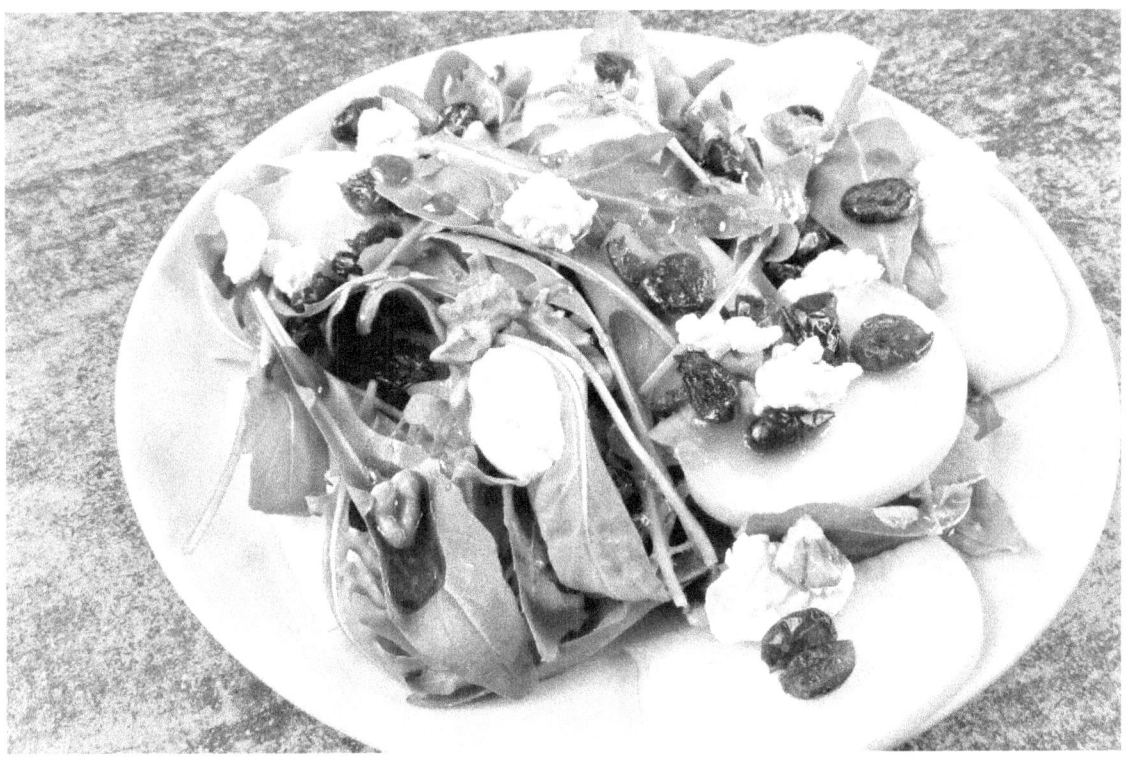

Arugula salad is a vibrant and peppery delight that excites the palate. This simple yet elegant dish features fresh arugula leaves tossed with cranberries, creating a harmonious balance of flavors.

Cooking time: 10 minutes

Servings: 1

Ingredients:

- 2 cups arugula leaves
- ¼ cup cranberries
- ¼ cup honey
- ¼ cup pecans
- 1 cup salad dressing

Instructions:

In a bowl, combine all ingredients together and mix well.

Serve with dressing.

38. Tuna Salad

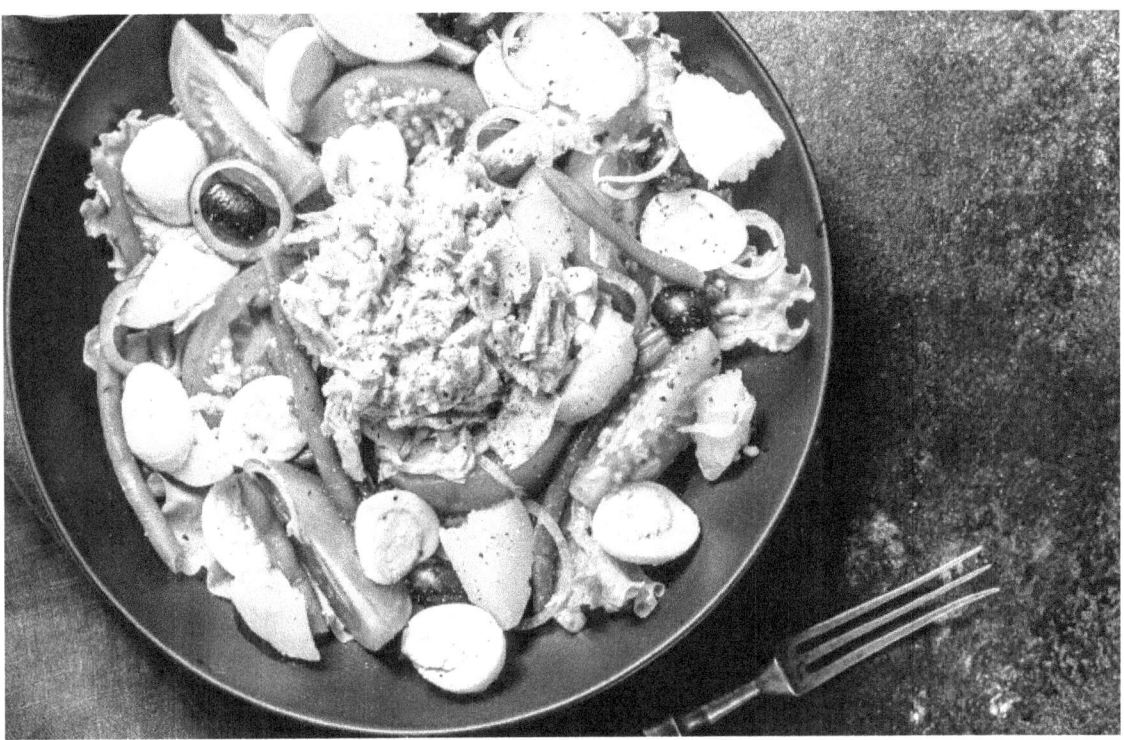

Tuna salad is a classic, no-fuss dish that's as versatile as it is delicious. Flaky tuna combines with mayo, celery, and other seasonings to create a creamy and satisfying concoction. Whether you scoop it onto a bed of greens, sandwich it between slices of bread, or serve it as a dip, tuna salad is a quick and easy meal that's loved by many.

Cooking time: 10 minutes

Servings: 1

Ingredients:

- 2 handful of salad leaves
- 1 can tuna
- Handful of coriander leaves
- 1 tablespoon olive oil

Instructions:

In a bowl, combine all ingredients together and mix well.

Serve with dressing.

39. Shrimp Salad

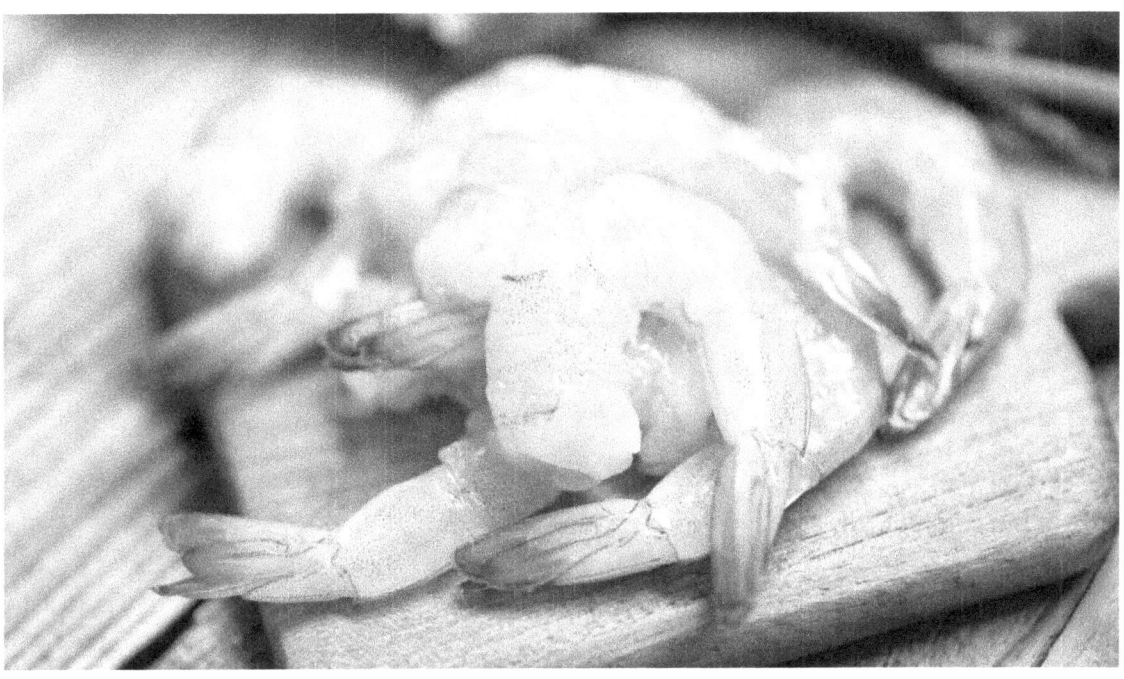

Shrimp salad is a delightful culinary experience that celebrates the ocean's bounty. Tender, succulent shrimp meet a medley of crisp vegetables and a zesty dressing, creating a refreshing and flavorful dish. This salad is a perfect balance of protein and veggies, making it a nutritious choice for any meal.

Cooking time: 10 minutes

Servings: 1

Ingredients:

- 1 lb. shrimp
- 2 tablespoons olive oil
- ¼ tsp paprika
- ¼ tsp cumin
- ¼ tsp turmeric
- 1 clove garlic
- ½ tsp salt

Instructions:

In a bowl, combine all ingredients together and mix well.

Serve with dressing.

40. Potato Salad

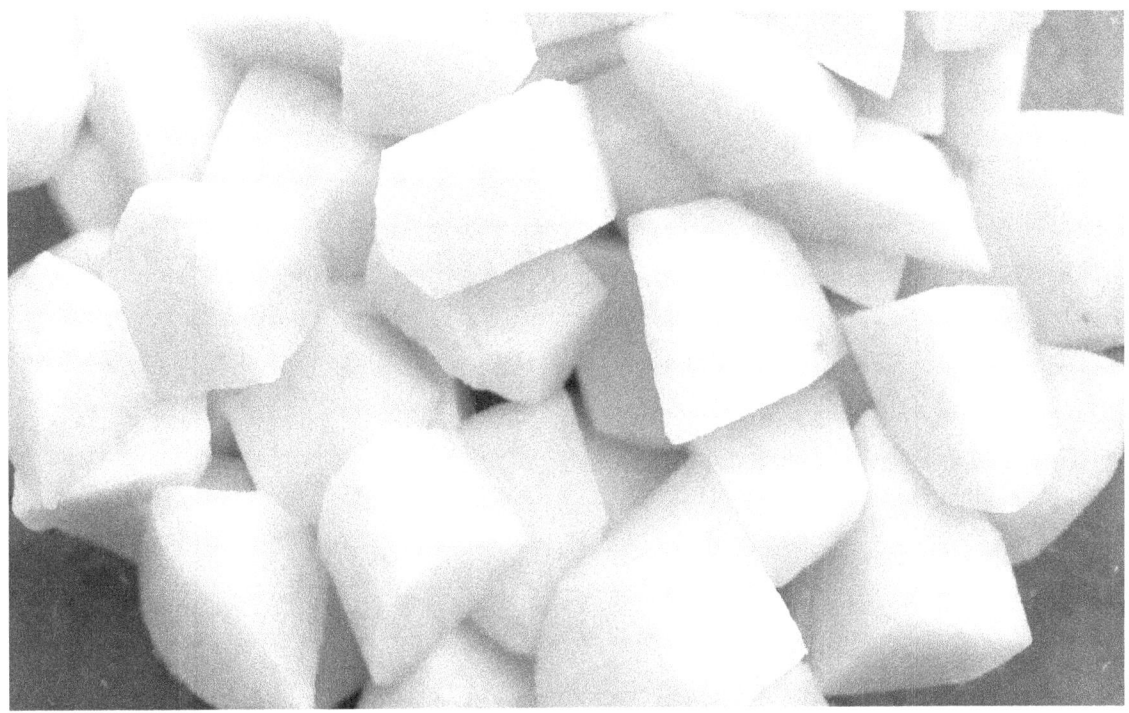

Potato salad is a timeless comfort food that's both hearty and satisfying. It's the quintessential comfort food that never goes out of style, offering a taste of home in every bite.

Cooking time: 10 minutes

Servings: 2

Ingredients:

- 4 cups white potato
- 1 pinch salt
- 2 tablespoons olive oil
- ¼ cup corn
- ½ cup black beans
- 2 tablespoons lemon juice

Instructions:

In a bowl, mix all ingredients and mix well.

Serve with dressing.

Chapter 5: Smoothies Recipes

41. Buttermilk Smoothie

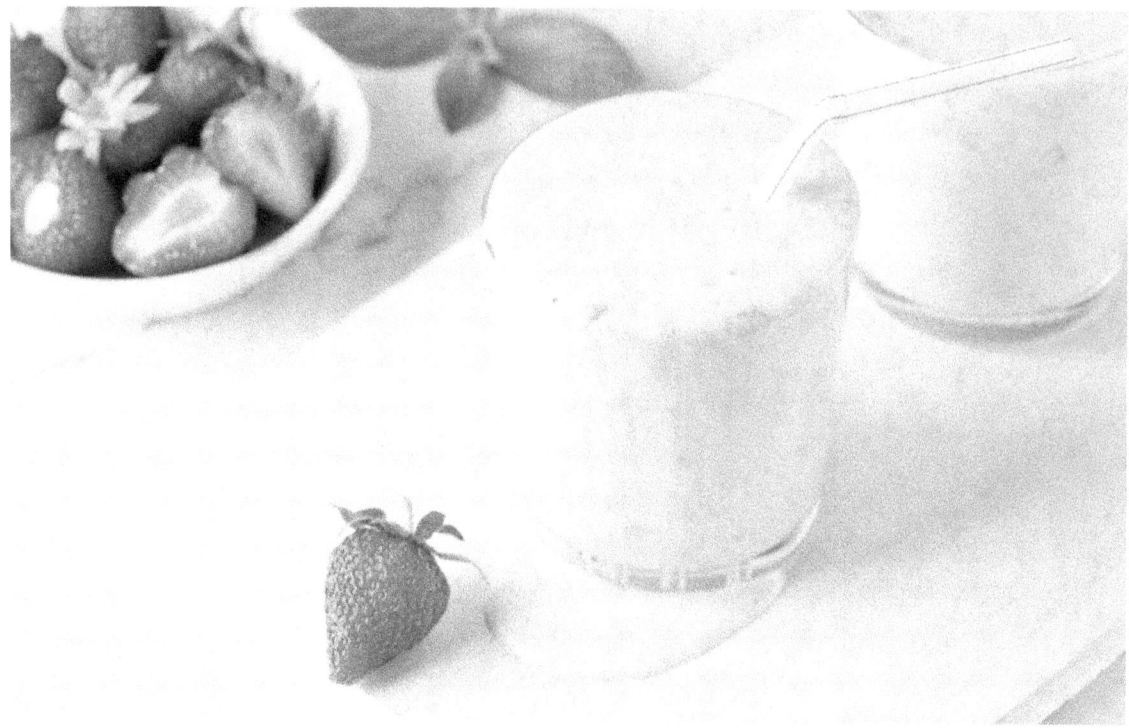

A buttermilk smoothie is a refreshing and unique twist on a classic favorite. This smoothie is not only delicious but also packed with probiotics, calcium, and vitamins, making it a wholesome choice for breakfast or a midday pick-me-up.

Cooking time: 10 minutes

Servings: 1

Ingredients:

- 1 cup strawberries
- 1 cup buttermilk
- 1 cup ice
- 1 tsp honey
- 1 tsp agave syrup

Instructions:

In a blender, place all ingredients and blend until smooth.

Pour smoothie in a glass and serve.

42. Pomegranate Smoothie

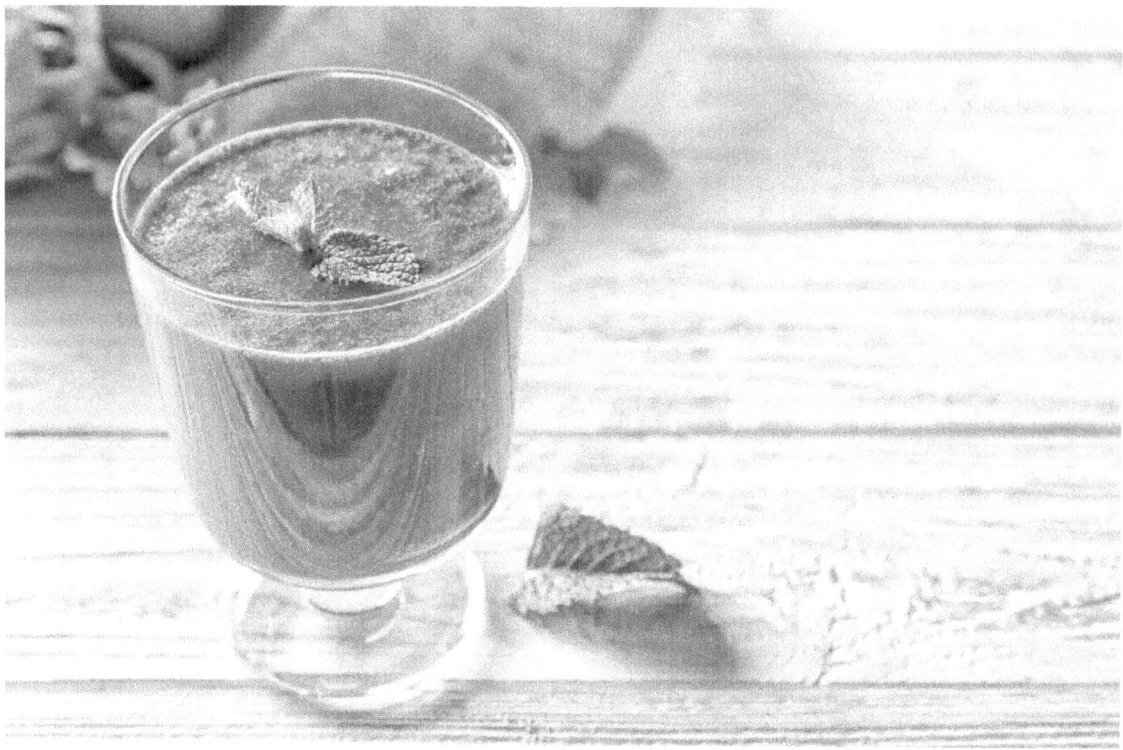

A pomegranate smoothie is a burst of vibrant flavor and health benefits in a glass. Juicy pomegranate seeds, blended with yogurt or your favorite base, create a refreshing and tangy concoction. Packed with antioxidants and vitamins, it's a nutritious choice that supports heart health and boosts your immune system.

Cooking time: 10 minutes

Servings: 1

Ingredients:

- 1 cup pomegranate juice
- ¼ cup vanilla yogurt
- 3 cooked beets
- ¼ cup grapefruit juice
- 1 tablespoon honey
- 1 cup ice

Instructions:

In a blender, place all ingredients and blend until smooth.

Pour smoothie in a glass and serve.

43. Parsley & Pineapple Smoothie

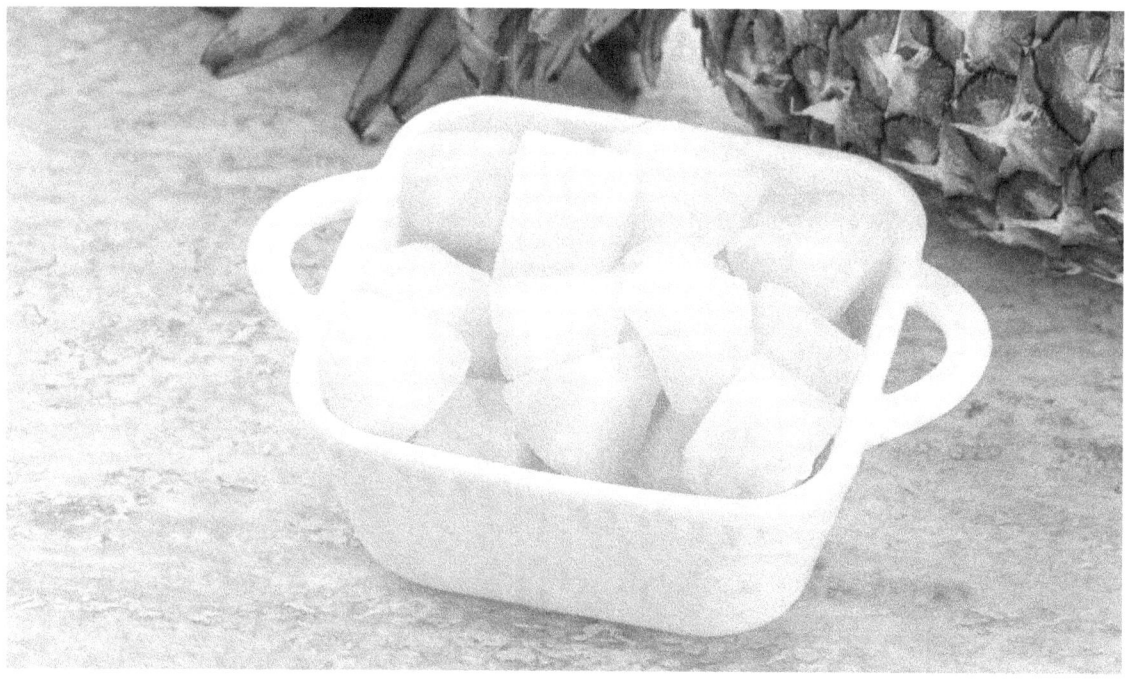

The parsley and pineapple smoothie is a green powerhouse with a tropical twist. This vibrant smoothie is loaded with vitamins, minerals, and antioxidants from the parsley, while the pineapple adds a zing of tropical flavor.

Cooking time: 15 minutes

Servings: 4

Ingredients:

- 1 banana
- 1 cup pineapple
- ¼ cup parsley
- 1 tsp chia seeds
- 1 cup ice

Instructions:

In a blender, place all ingredients and blend until smooth.

Pour smoothie in a glass and serve.

44. Mango & Watermelon Smoothie

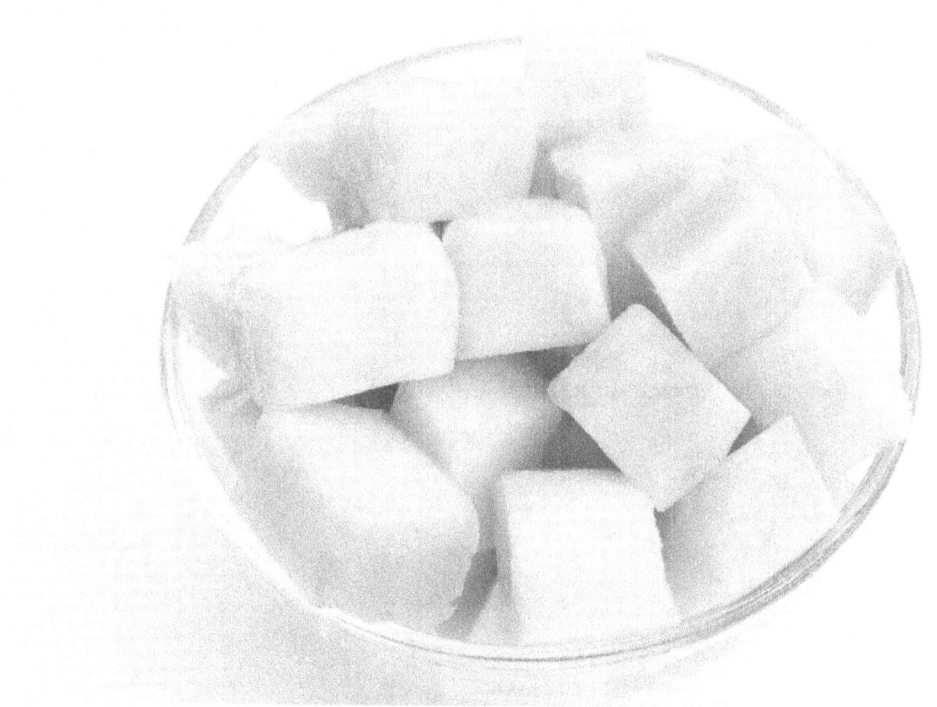

This smoothie is a taste of paradise in every sip, making it the perfect way to beat the summer heat and stay energized.

Cooking time: 10 minutes

Servings: 2

Ingredients:

- 2 mangoes
- ½ lb. watermelon
- 1-2 tablespoons mint leaves
- 1 tray ice cube

Instructions:

In a blender, place all the ingredients and blend until smooth.

Pour smoothie into a glass and serve.

45. Mango Smoothie

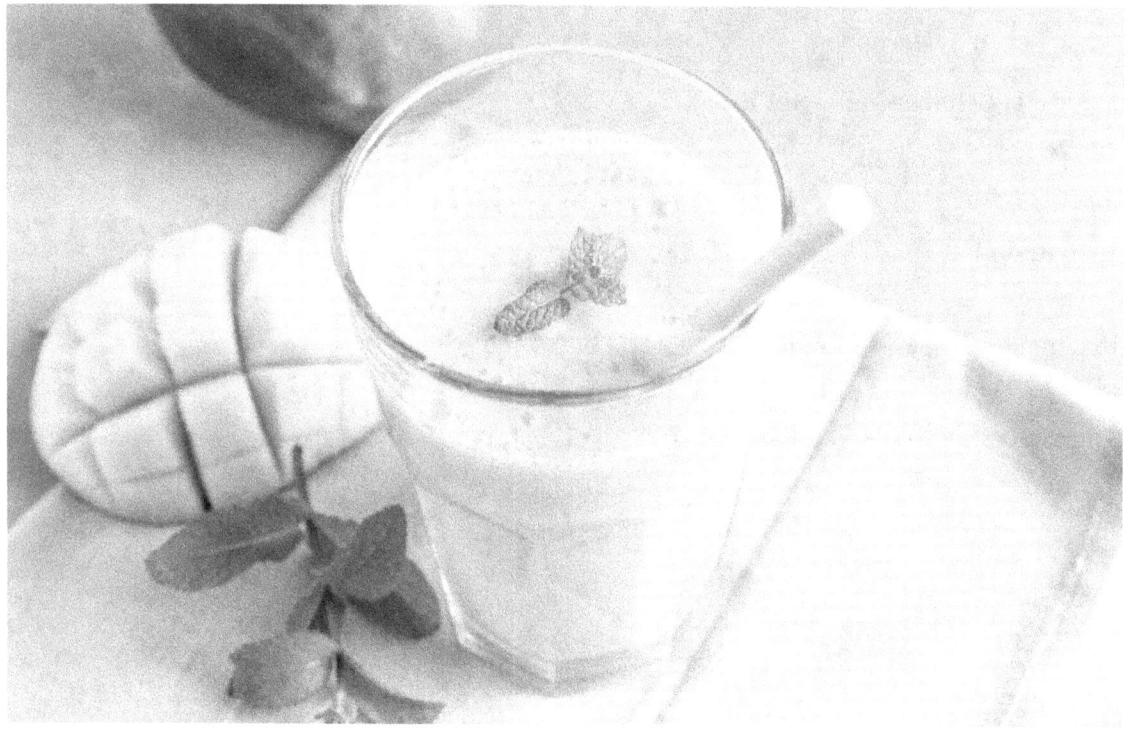

Quench your thirst and support your lymphatic system with our refreshing Mango Smoothie. Packed with vitamin C, antioxidants, and anti-inflammatory properties, this tropical delight is a delicious way to combat lymphedema.

Cooking time: 10 minutes

Servings: 1

Ingredients:

- 1 cup orange juice
- ¼ cup vanilla yogurt
- 1 cup mango
- 1 carrot
- 1 cup ice

Instructions:

In a blender, place all ingredients and blend until smooth.

Pour smoothie in a glass and serve.

46. Papaya Smoothie

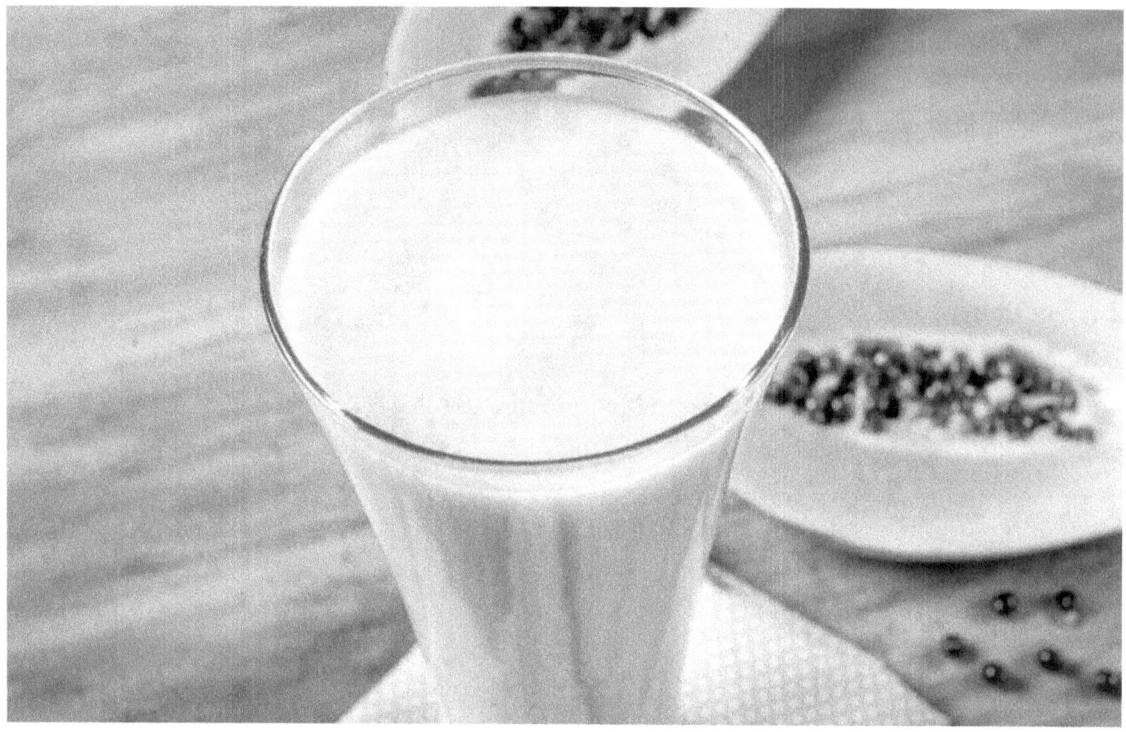

Enjoy a refreshing papaya smoothie that not only tantalizes your taste buds but also promotes well-being. It's a delicious and nutritious treat suitable for everyone, any time of the day.

Cooking time: 10 minutes

Servings: 1

Ingredients:

- 1 cup coconut flakes
- ½ cup papaya
- 1 tablespoon goji berries
- 1 tablespoon chia seeds
- 1 banana
- 1 cup ice

Instructions:

In a blender, place all ingredients and blend until smooth.

Pour smoothie in a glass and serve.

47. Peanut Butter Smoothie

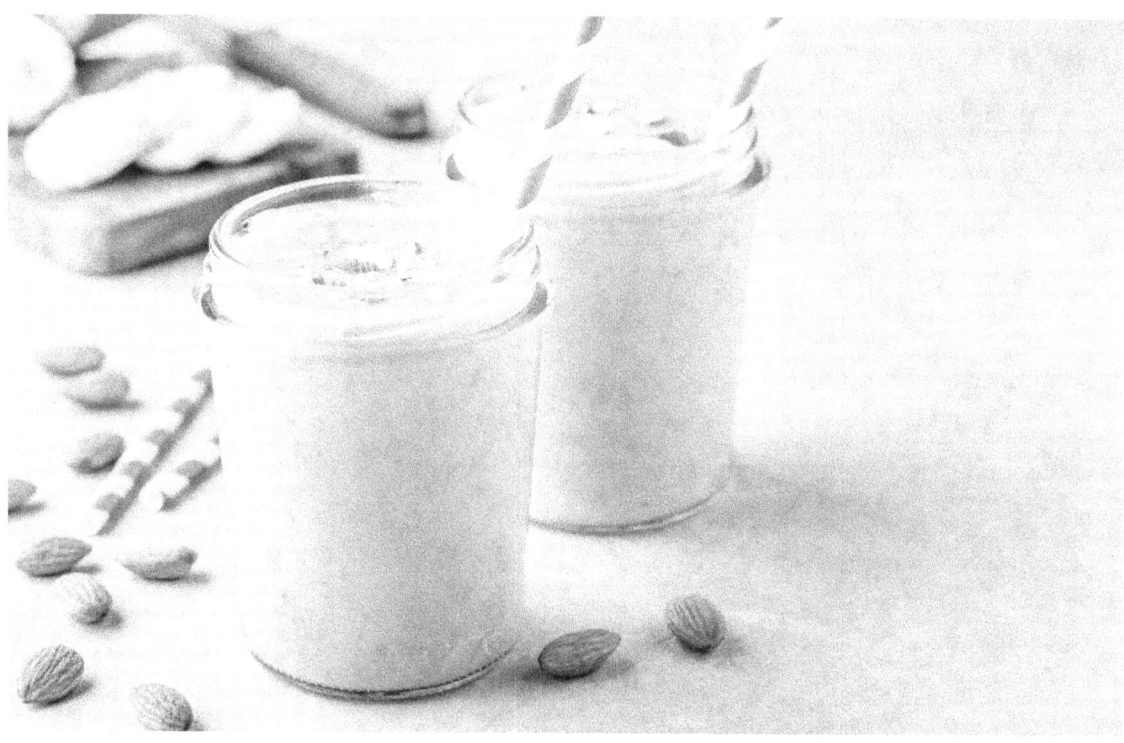

This creamy concoction combines the nutty goodness of peanut butter with the benefits of bananas and Greek yogurt. Packed with protein, potassium, and essential nutrients, it's a perfect choice for a quick breakfast or post-workout snack.

Cooking time: 10 minutes

Servings: 1

Ingredients:

- 1 banana
- 1 cup milk
- 2 tablespoons peanut butter
- 1 cup ice

Instructions:

In a blender place all ingredients and blend until smooth

Pour smoothie in a glass and serve

48. Creamsicle Smoothie

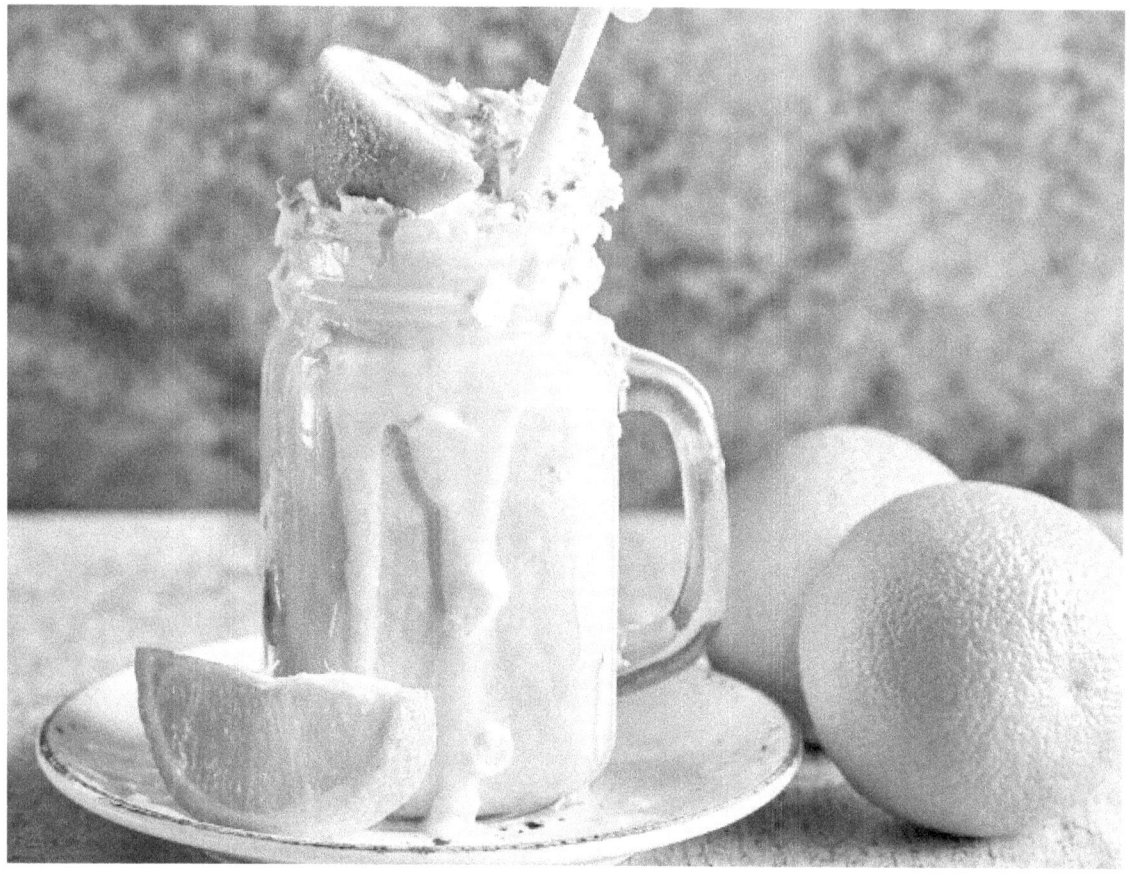

This smoothie is a perfect choice for anyone looking to boost their immune system and satisfy their taste buds. Whether you're managing lymphedema or simply want a refreshing, guilt-free snack, this smoothie is a must-try for all.

Cooking time: 10 minutes

Servings: 1

Ingredients:

- 2 cups mango
- 1 carrot
- 1 tablespoon apple cider vinegar
- 1 tsp lemon juice
- 1 cup coconut milk
- 1 tsp honey

Instructions:

In a blender, place all ingredients and blend until smooth.

Pour smoothie in a glass and serve.

49. Berry Smoothie

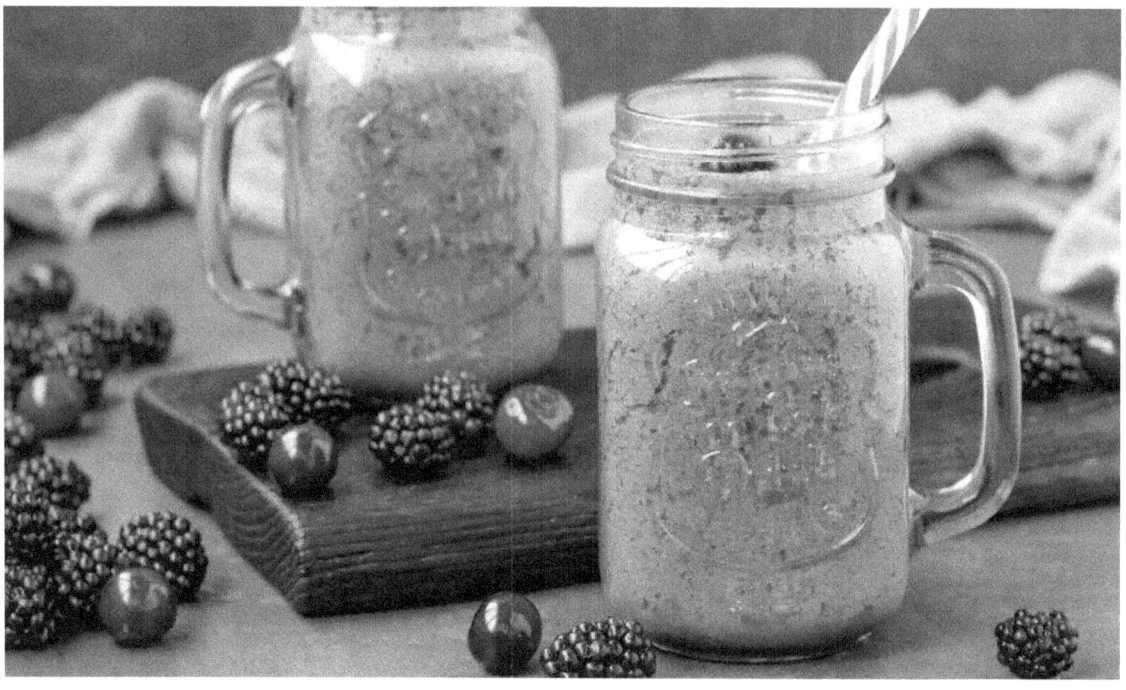

This Berry Smoothie is a delicious and nutritious treat that's perfect for everyone. Packed with a medley of fresh berries, it's a refreshing way to boost your health.

Cooking time: 10 minutes

Servings: 1

Ingredients:

- 1 banana
- 4 cups pineapple juice
- 1 cup ice
- 4 oz. blueberries
- 4 oz. blackberries
- 1 tablespoon honey

Instructions:

In a blender, place all ingredients and blend until smooth.

Pour smoothie in a glass and serve.

50. Carrot Smoothie

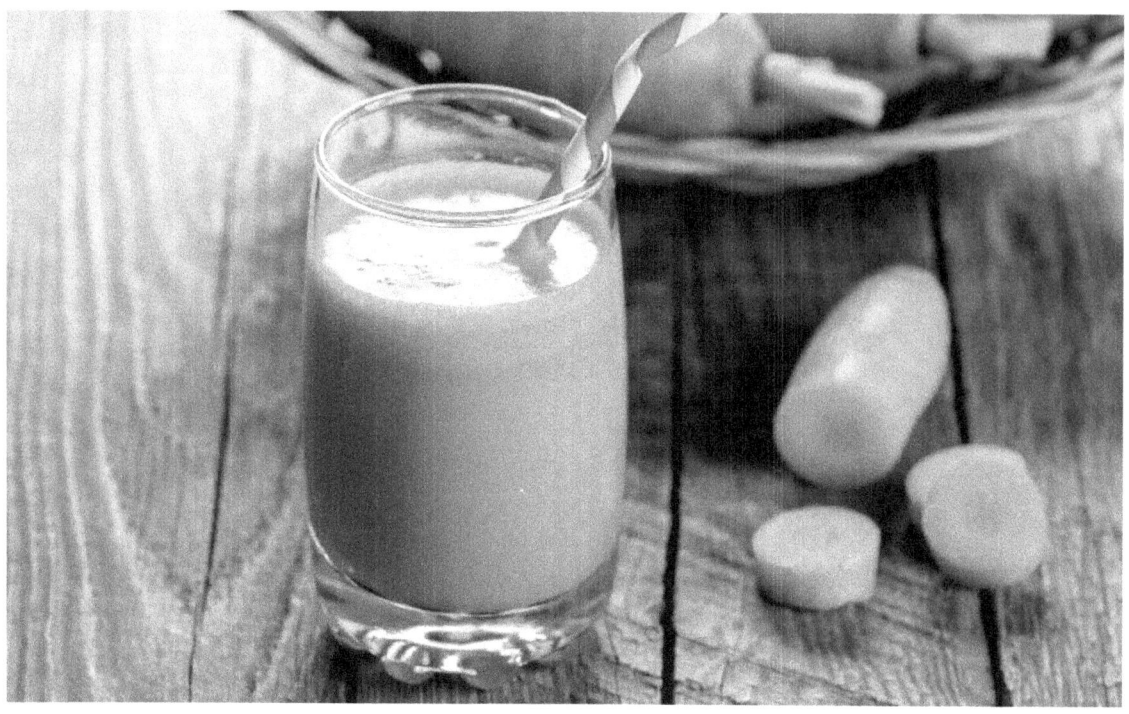

Revitalize your day with our refreshing carrot smoothie, a delightful blend of fresh carrots, pineapple, and a hint of ginger. Packed with anti-inflammatory properties, this tasty concoction is a game-changer for lymphedema management.

Cooking time: 10 minutes

Servings: 2

Ingredients:

- 1 carrot
- 2 oranges
- 1-2 tablespoons mint leaves
- 1 tray ice cube

Instructions:

In a blender, place all the ingredients and blend until smooth.

Pour smoothie into a glass and serve.

Conclusion

Thank you for reaching the end of this book. Remember that a lymphedema-friendly diet is just one piece of the puzzle, and it should be complemented by other aspects of lymphedema management, such as exercise, skincare, and proper medical guidance. But with this cookbook in your hands, you now have the tools to create tasty and nutritious meals that align with your lymphatic health goals.

We hope these 50 super tasty recipes will inspire you to embark on a delicious and nutritious journey while managing lymphedema. Whether you're a seasoned cook or a beginner in the kitchen, there's something in this cookbook for everyone.

Thank you for choosing to prioritize your health and well-being, and we wish you many enjoyable and satisfying meals ahead on your lymphedema journey. May each bite be a step toward a healthier and happier you.

Thank You

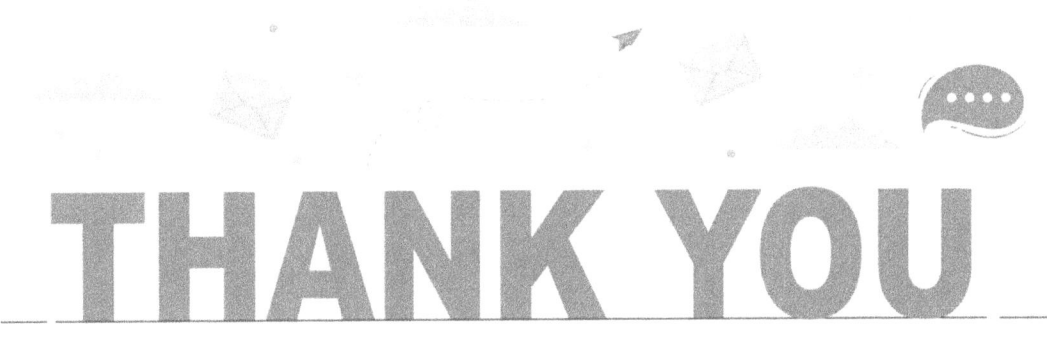

The gratitude I feel for your purchase of my book cannot be expressed in words. Each sale shows me that individuals are benefiting from my experiences and knowledge. Becoming a writer was a decision I made because it allows me to share my skills and expertise with others.

Out of the numerous books available, you chose mine, which is extremely special to me. I have no doubt that the information presented in the book will be useful and informative for you.

Please remember to leave feedback once you've finished reading the book. Every piece of feedback, no matter how small, is invaluable to me in creating even better books. I listen carefully to my readers and take their suggestions into account when developing new content. Your honest feedback will be incorporated into my next books.

Thank you once again for your support.

Alain Duke